Autophagy:

Unlock the Human Body's Power for Self Healing, Anti Aging and Weight Loss

Levi Wood

before using any of the suggested remedies, techniques, or information in this book.

Upon using the contents and information contained in this book, you agree to hold harmless the Author from and against any damages, costs, and expenses, including any legal fees potentially resulting from the application of any of the information provided by this book. This disclaimer applies to any loss, damages or injury caused by the use and application, whether directly or indirectly, of any advice or information presented, whether for breach of contract, tort, negligence, personal injury, criminal intent, or under any other cause of action.

You agree to accept all risks of using the information presented inside this book.

You agree that by continuing to read this book, where appropriate and/or necessary, you shall consult a professional (including but not limited to your doctor, attorney, or financial advisor or such other advisor as needed) before using any of the suggested remedies, techniques, or information in this book.

Table of Content

Chapter 1:
What is Autophagy?

Introduction

The progress of science enables us to understand nature more than before. Science tells us that nature is in a continuous energetic movement between creation (synthesis) and destruction (degradation). Unlike man-made machines, nature maintains an equilibrium between synthesis and degradation. The degradation process was known to involve those compounds and organisms outside the cell or the body, like in the digestion of food. However, recent scientific research disclosed that "digestion" can occur inside the cell as well. The cell has evolutionarily developed a unique system for renewing itself and creating new ones. This system is responsible for the turnover over of proteins, small organs, and various cell structures. This system is discovered by a Belgian scientist called Christian de Duve who give this system the name of "autophagy."

The Discovery of Autophagy

In the mid-1950, an organelle (a small specialized cellular compartment) was found to contain enzymes that are involved in the digestion of cellular proteins and small organs within the cells. This specialized cellular compartment was called lysosomes (from the Greek word "lyso" meaning *destruction* and *"some"* meaning body)[1]. Lysosomes act as a workspace for the degradation of cellular components.

In 1963, Christian de Duve, a Belgian biochemist scientist, assigned the term *autophagy* to the process of destruction of cell components lysosomes[2], [3]. The name, again, is derived from the Greek word "autos" meaning *"self"* and "phagy" meaning *"to eat"*. C. De Duve found a large number of cellular components and whole organelles inside the lysosomes. He described that the cell seems to have a strategy to deliver large *cargo* to the lysosomes. C. De Duve discovered another structure involved in *cargo* delivery. The newly discovered structures were called auto phagosome (from old Greek *"autophagy"* meaning *"self-devouring"* and "Kytos" meaning *"hollow."*

In 1990, Yoshinori Ohsumi carried out a series of intelligent experiments on baker's yeast. Yoshinori succeeded in identifying the genes essential for autophagy. His discovery was a breakthrough in the science of autophagy. Ohsumi, induced gene mutation in the yeast that induced autophagy. The mutant cells showed disrupted autophagy at different stages of the process depending on gene mutation. This technique enabled Ohsumi and the following scientists to identify autophagy genes (ATG) and the proteins encoded by these genes. Now we understand that autophagy is carried out by a cascade of proteins and complexes each of which is responsible for controlling a separate stage of autophagy series process. Now, we understand to a greater extent the mechanisms underlying autophagy in yeast. We expect that a similar process takes place in mammals as well- including humans.

Chapter 2:
How autophagy works

Autophagy is a term that refers to the process of degradation of the cell components by lysosomes. There are three types of autophagy inside the cell including macro-autophagy, microautophagy, and chaperone-mediated autophagy. We usually use autophagy to refer to the macro-autophagy process.

The World of Autophagy

The cell of humans is composed of the central nucleus and cytoplasm. Cytoplasm refers to all material components within the cell that is enclosed by the cell membrane except the nucleus. The cytoplasm is composed of cytosol, a gel-like material, and organelles, the small cell structures such as mitochondria (the powerhouse), endoplasmic reticulum (a continuous membrane system), and ribosomes (protein factory). Cytoplasm contains, also, lipid droplets and vacuoles. Most cellular activities take place within the cytoplasm.

It is clear that autophagy constitutes several successive steps including sequestration, degradation, and amino acid or peptide generation. These different steps have different functions in different cellular situations. Considering the role of autophagy in stress, anti-aging, anti-microbial, and tumor suppression, the different steps enables autophagy to perform multiple functions for the benefit of the cell [4].

The autophagy process starts by enclosing a portion of the cytoplasm within the autophagosome. Autophagosome is a membranous structure. The outer membrane of the autophagosome fuses with the lysosome. The lysosome contains hydrolytic enzymes that degrade proteins and other organelles. The degradation products are building units such as amino acids and fatty acids. The cell uses these building units to build new cell proteins or organelles that are necessary for the cell function.

Unlike macroautophagy (also referred to as autophagy), microautophagy also knows as lesser-knows self-eating, refers to the direct lysosomal fusion with the cytoplasmic cargo. Lysosomes engulf the cytoplasmic material without the formation of auto phagosomes. The cytoplasmic cargo invaginates within the membrane of the lysosomes. The sequestrated material is now subject to the hydrolytic effect of the lysosomal enzymes. Micro autophagy pathway is activated at the time of starvation stress, nitrogen deprivation, and after rapamycin therapy [5].

Chaperone-mediated autophagy (CMA) is a selective pathway acting on soluble cytosolic proteins that are delivered to lysosomes directly without the formation of auto phagosomes [6].

We conclude that autophagy is a process of degradation of large molecules that are either modified, surplus, or damaged as well as other organelles within the cells. This complex process involves the destructive enzymes (hydrolytic) within the lysosomes[7]. In fact, autophagy is used to refer to any destructive process inside the cells that involves the delivery of cytoplasmic cargo to the lysosomes.

The Processes and Types of Autophagy

Triggering of Autophagy

Lack of the essential nutrients in the cell is a strong trigger for autophagy to start up. Proteins are the most important cell nutrients the deficiency of which strongly triggers autophagy to work. It has been found that other nutrients play the same triggering role such as carbon, amino acids, nucleic acids, and sulfate. However, their triggering effect is lagging behind that of proteins [8].

How the cell comes to know that the amino acids are lacking is not well identified. Recently, the endocrine role has been emphasized as the signaling process for the cell to activate autophagy. Liver autophagy, for examples, has demonstrated suppression of autophagy with high insulin level. insulin is secreted when one eats and the sugar level in blood increases. On the other hand, liver autophagy is enhanced with the increase of glucagon in blood. Glucagon in insulin counter hormone. It increases during the periods of hunger sensed by a low glucose level. Other autophagy signaling process includes growth factors such as interleukin 3 (IL3) [9].

The signaling process of amino acids, insulin, and growth factors are mediated by several mechanisms including the mammalian target of rapamycin (mTOR). The inhibition of mTOR induces autophagy. Therefore, mTOR has become the target for therapeutic trials to stimulate autophagy medically. Rapamycin and CCI-779, the inhibitors for mTOR, have shown great implications in the treatment of clinical conditions by activation of autophagy [10].

Formation of Auto phagosomes

Auto phagosome formation is the first step in autophagy, the cytoplasmic constituents and cell organelles are sequestrated by a special membrane called phagophore (isolation membrane). The phagophore is elongated to complete the sequestration process and auto phagosome is thus formed its double membrane structure.

Fluorescence microscopy has identified a certain site in the cell as punctate spot close to vacuolar membranes. It has been found that autophagy starts from this site. The punctate spots shown by fluorescence microscopy represent the accumulation of autophagy-related proteins (Atg). These proteins are designated in numbers. The participating role of each protein has not been clearly identified. However, Atg8 is found to mediate tethering and partial fusion of liposomes. This fusion process was suggested as a possibility for the elongation of the phagophore membrane, hence the formation of auto phagosomes [11].

Autophagy Degradation

Degradation is the following step in the autophagy process. The already formed auto phagosomes fuse with a lysosome. The fusion of lysosome and auto phagosome form a single structure called autophagolysosomes. The lysosome contains lipase-like enzymes designated as Atg15, Atg5, Cvt17. These enzymes degrade the inner membrane of the auto phagosome as well as the cytoplasm-derived material inside the auto phagosome. Moreover, endosomes participate in the degradation process by providing the auto phagosomes the needed machinery for lysosome fusion. The autophagy degradation structures are called collectively autophagic vacuoles [12].

The Recycling Process

The final process is the export of the degradation material to the cytosol for reuse and recycling. This process is very useful for protein turnover. The cells can use the degradation products e.g. amino acids to synthesize new proteins and protein-based structure. However, the contribution of autophagy in the turnover of carbs and fat has not been identified yet [13]. It has been postulated that the released amino acids are reused to synthesize new proteins that are useful for the cell to cope with stress, infection, or tumor suppression. Therefore, the degradation process of autophagy contributes to the renewal of the cell keeping its vitality and participating in its longevity.

The Promising Outcome of Autophagy

The recent discoveries underscore the process of protein turnover, recycling of cell content, and scavenging the aged structures. Moreover, the deep understanding of how autophagy function and is controlled elaborated the important role of autophagy in various physiological processes.

Autophagy and starvation

Autophagy is involved in the adaptation of the organism to starvation. Starvation represents a challenge, *stress,* to cell survival. During starvations, the energy and nutrients of the cells are consumed up threatening cell vivacity. Autophagy is an essential mechanism for providing cells in stress with fuel for energy. Autophagy provides the cells with building blocks for renewal of cellular components. In essence, autophagy degrades the non-essential proteins and organelles and provide the cells with amino acids and fatty acids. These are building blocks that can be used by the cells to synthesize essential components for challenging stress including starvation.

Autophagy and infections

Autophagy helps our bodies to respond effectively to infections. Autophagy is essential in eliminating the invading organisms. The invading bacteria or viruses are engulfed by the phagocytes and delivered to the lysosomes for degradation.

Autophagy and development

During embryonic development, the cells are subject to tremendous turnover. The embryo is in a continuous turnover with the creation of new cells and degradation of other cells resulting in the development of the fetal organs. Autophagy act as a programmed cell death mechanism. The no-more-needed cells are destroyed by autophagy to make room for new cells to develop or to eliminate a no-more-needed organ. Moreover, autophagy plays an important role in cell differentiation. That is to say, the cells transform into more specialized and functioning cells.

Autophagy and aging

Furthermore, abnormality in activation or suppression of autophagy can lead to disease. It has been noticed that autophagy is associated with the development of age-related diseases such as neurodegenerative diseases and muscle atrophy (decay). This happens when autophagy wanes off by the advance of age. It has been proved that disrupted autophagy is strongly associated with Parkinson's disease, type 2 diabetes, and atherosclerosis. The risk of these diseases is known to increase with the advance of age.

__Autophagy and fasting__

It has been found that autophagy is halted (inhibited) by feeding and activated during the process of fasting between meals [14], [15]. After 48 hours of starvation, 30-40% of proteins in the liver would be degraded [16], [17]. Fasting initiates the rise of glucagon hormone, the opponent to insulin hormone. The rise of glucagon hormone synthesis activates the process of autophagy. Then, autophagy performs two important functions. The first function is the removal of the old, aged, and abnormally folded proteins. The aged cell structures and organelles are disposed of as well. It is the scavenging part of autophagy. The second mechanism is the stimulation of growth hormone. The growth hormone boosts the synthesis of new cell components and new cells. Growth hormones signal the renewal of our body as a whole. Activation of autophagy by fasting helps provide the cell and hence the body, by nutrients to keep vital cellular process. Remarkably, autograph, self-digestion, is rising as a prominent biological process that promotes the health and longevity of our cells[3]. In essence, the old and cultural tradition of fasting is now understood in the scientific lens as a process by which the body makes a new carpet from the old one. The ancient tradition of fasting has long been attributed to health and healing sacred practices. It has been believed that renewal of the body cells and organelles help challenge aging and halt or prolong the process of body decay.

Autophagy and Skin Aging

Young skin is loaded with collagen protein that preserves skin integrity. Loss of skin integrity is the result of a lack of collagen protein. Fibroblasts are the cells responsible for the synthesis of collagen. With the advance of age, fibroblasts stop synthesizing collagen rendering the skin look *old*. It has been discovered that autophagy recycles the fibroblast cell structure and creates new ones. Deficient autophagy by aging leads to the accumulation of unfolded proteins, old structures, and other waste products. The fibroblasts become packed with wastes that grind collagen product to a halt. The reduction of collagen formation by fibroblast leads the skin to look fragile and wrinkled. When we activate autophagy, by either fasting or certain pharmaco-therapeutic agents, collagen production is resumed, and skin keeps young.

Chapter 3:
Autophagy in Health and Disease

Autophagy in Health

Autophagy and stress

It has been found that autophagy is activated as a response to various types of stresses. When our bodies face famine (food deprivation), lack of the needed growth factors, or decrease of oxygen coming into the body, autophagy is the adaptive mechanism that our bodies adapt to face these stressful conditions.

The autophagy degradation produces free amino acids and fatty acids that constitute the structure of both proteins and fat respectively. Then, our bodies use these products to synthesize new proteins that are mandatory for the cells to face and adapt to stress. The molecular basis for the turnover of proteins by autophagy process has been recently identified in studies conducted on yeast [18].

Moreover, autophagy helps supply cells with energy at a time of stress when the resources for energy are lacking. The produced amino acids and fatty acids liberated from the autophagy process fuel the Krebs' cycle. Krebs' cycle is a series of chemical reactions that produce energy for the cell. In case of stress, the main fuel for Krebs' cycle i.e. glucose, fat, and proteins are lacking. Therefore, the deficiency of this nutrient at time of stress threatens cell survival. The crucial role of autophagy is degradation of non-essential proteins and fat into amino acids and fatty acids to fuel Krebs' cycle that generates adenosine triphosphate (ATP), the energy molecule of the cell [19]. The generated ATP molecules supply the cells with energy at the time of stress and preserve cells from decay [20]. So, during nutrient stress autophagy plays an essential pro-survival role for keeping cells functioning.

Studies on animals have clarified the critical physiological role of autophagy in the mobilization of intracellular energy resources to generate the needed chemical compounds (substrates) for the cells and organism. In addition to nutrient starvation, lack of growth factor signaling for nutrient uptake leads to a decrease of the needed substrates inside the cells and hence, activation of autophagy survival process [21]. Moreover, when the cell has increased demand for metabolites at any particular time, autophagy is autonomously activated to provide the cell with the needed substrates [22].

Autophagy as a housekeeper of cells

It has been proved that autophagy performs important functions inside the cell. Autophagy help eliminate proteins and organelles with defects in their structure that hinder their proper function. Autophagy destroys abnormal proteins, thus preventing the accumulation of abnormal proteins within the cell. Last but not least, the intracellular pathogens (harmful materials) are also removed by autophagy. Therefore, autophagy plays a scavenging role inside the cells to rid the cell of non-functioning and harmful proteins and pathogens. This scavenging role is expressed as cellular housekeeping function.

The scavenging role of autophagy plays a critical role in protecting the cell against aging, cancer, and neurodegenerative diseases. Autophagy, the housekeeper, protects the cell from infections as well.

The housekeeper, autophagy, prevent accumulation of altered or abnormally folded proteins inside the cells. On the other hand, failure of protein turnover leads to accumulation of protein aggregates. The impairment of protein turnover causes damage to proteins. The damaged proteins attach to ubiquitin compound that changes how the proteins function within the cell. The attached proteins to ubiquitin tend to aggregate inside the cell

[23]. The aggregated proteins could be harmful to the cell. Alzheimer's disease is suggested to be due to the disruption of the autophagy process leading to accumulation of protein aggregate within the cells [24]. It is the function of autophagy to remove such types of protein. It is what the housekeeper for.

Moreover, autophagy is capable of eliminating the disrupted organelles such as mitochondria (energy generator organelles), peroxisomes (micro bodies for catabolism of long chain fatty acids), and endoplasmic reticulum (an interconnected network of membrane-enclosed sacs). Certain signals for recognizing selectively damaged or excessive (superfluous) organelles have been identified. These signals initiate autophagy to eliminate these organelles from the cell [25], [26]. It has been proven that defective autophagy to eliminate surplus or damaged mitochondria increases the tendency of development of cardio degenerative diseases [27]. Regular elimination of mitochondria reduces oxidative stress and hence tissue damage. This process reduces cancer signaling process resulting in suppression of cancer [28].

Autophagy as a genome guardian

Autophagy is implicated in the protection of DNA and preserve its integrity within the nucleolus [29]. DNA refers to deoxyribonucleic acid; it carries genetic information and instructions for cell growth, development, and various cell functions. we recall that autophagy plays an important role in energy homeostasis and control of protein and organelles. These known functions are suggested to act as protective mechanisms against DNA disruption.

Autophagy acts as a guardian to DNA through several mechanisms. Autophagy helps prevent damage of DNA checkpoint or repair proteins. The DNA checkpoint disables cell division (mitosis) till DNA is fully replicated or damaged DNA is fully repaired. Otherwise, the cell is threatened with death (apoptosis) after cell division [30]. Therefore, autophagy is vital for cell survival and homeostasis.

The function of autophagy in the removal of excessive mitochondria from the interior of the cell guarding against excessive production of reactive oxygen species by these mitochondria [31]. The reactive oxygen species are chemically reactive compounds containing oxygen in a tremendously active form [32]. When these species increase within the cell, they become destructive to cell structures including the DNA genome. Here comes the role of autophagy to scavenge mitochondria, reduces the active species and protects DNA genome [33].

The protective function of autophagy for the DNA genome is carried out through different another mechanism. The net result is maintaining the integrity and function of the DNA genome and consequently cell survival. Any factor that disrupts the process of autophagy would lead to either cell death or the development of human disorders such as premature aging, cancer, and degenerative diseases [28], [33].

Autophagy in cell life and death decision (apoptosis)

Introduction

Cell death has been extensively studied for understanding the mechanism of the development of disease and its progress. The interesting implications of such studies on autophagy cell death are the discovery of new drug generation that is able to beat for cancer and degenerative disorders. There are different pathways and mechanisms of cell death. Apoptosis and autophagy play an interlacing role in cell death. We have talked about the cytoprotective mechanism of autophagy in the previous sections. The following section will talk about apoptosis, a cell death mechanism, and its interconnection with autophagy for cell death.

In organisms like humans -us -the number of cells in our organ is regulated by "cell birth" and "cell death." It seems that the cell "kill" itself after receiving a certain signal. The received signal activates a cell program naturally impeded within the cell genomes, the so-called programmed cell death (PCD). It is also called apoptosis (a Greek word meaning "falling off," resembling falling leaves in fall) [34]. The apoptosis is massive among cells in certain organ leaving us with a question about the purpose of this massive cell death. Apoptosis is responsible for the disappearance of the no-more-needed cells or organ in the course of the organism development. In other cases, cell death optimizes the cell number in the organ. However, the final answer has not been reached yet [35].

Apoptosis is a designated term to the principle of cell self-destruction. In apoptosis, proteins named caspases are activated. These proteins destroy the cellular components of cell survival. They, also, activates enzymes that destroy the DNA genome inside the nucleus [36], [37].

Autophagy and apoptosis

Autophagy and apoptosis can be either two independent mechanisms for cell death acting in parallel pathways or two complementary ways with one pathway influencing the other. Autophagy is activated when the cell is under stressful conditions. Activation of autophagy leads to scavenging of aged or damaged organelles leading to accumulation of autophagic vacuoles. The accumulation of these vacuoles is often attributed to the dying cell. This feature may represent the failure of the autophagy adaptive mechanism to keep the cell alive [38]. Autophagy occurs ahead of apoptosis. Therefore, increased activation of autophagy may signal apoptotic cell death. Autophagy itself can cause cell death with the formation of the destructive bodies, auto phagosomes. This contradictive function is supported by the similarity between the outcome of both autophagy and apoptosis both in the morphology and biochemical characteristics [39]. Autophagy generates auto phagosomes that are similar in function and outcome to the apoptotic bodies generated by apoptosis [40]

The interplay between the two pathways leads scientists to believe that there is a "cross-talk" between autophagy and apoptosis [41]. This "cross-talk" process would determine the final outcome of the autophagy whether it will be cytoprotective i.e. protect the cell from facing death or herald cell death by apoptosis [42]. The "cross-talk" has been shown to be modulated by regulatory genes. The regulatory genes designated as p53, Atg5, and Bcl-2 has been believed to share with common pathways. Therefore, the final cell fate is affected by activation or inhibition of these genes by specific signaling pathways [43].

The interplay between autophagy and apoptosis have serious implications. It has been found that autophagy and apoptosis are involved in the etiology and/ or the development of neurodegenerative disorders [44]. Scientific research has found that autophagy activated by the stress of endoplasmic reticulum (ER) and misfolding of proteins has serious implication in the development of kidney disorders. Autophagy-mediated kidney disorder is characterized by the appearance of albumin in urine. Autophagy has been shown is the degenerative kidney disorders including acute kidney injury, chronic kidney injury, diabetic kidney disease, and other degenerative glomerular disorders [45]. Last but not least, the complex interplay between autophagy and apoptosis in liver cells determine the progress of liver diseases [36].

Autophagy in disease

In this section, we will discuss in detail how autophagy, the self-destructive mechanism, impact the etiology, development, and progress of diseases. The implications involve almost every organ on our bodies.

<u>Neurodegenerative diseases</u>

What are neurodegenerative diseases? Neurodegenerative disease is a generic term including a wide range of clinical conditions that involve the brain cells (neurons) in our nervous system. The nervous system includes the brain and the spinal cord. Normally, the brain cells are not reproduced or replaced. Therefore, our body is unable to replace the damaged neurons or reproduce new ones. Extensive damage to the neurons or death of brain or nerve cells causes serious and incurable disability. The patient may suffer problems in movement (ataxia) or mental functions (dementia). For example, neurodegenerative diseases include Alzheimer's disease, Parkinson's disease, and Huntington's disease. The list would be longer to be mentioned in full in this context.

The role of autophagy in neurodegenerative diseases: it was noticed that auto phagosomes accumulate in the neurons of the afflicted patients. Recent studies have proved that the accumulation of auto phagosomes is the result of extensive activation of autophagy. Autophagy activation is a useful physiological response to protect the neurons against the disease. Failure of auto phagosomes in degrading the contents would lead to their accumulation within the neurons resulting in cell damage. The latter process is observed in patients with Alzheimer's disease [46].

Another process that contributes to the development of neurodegenerative diseases is the accumulation of aggregate-prone mutant proteins. They are abnormal misfielded toxic proteins that tend to accumulate in the neurons causing their damage. These types of pathological proteins (hence the name proteopathy) have been proved to be responsible for the development and progression of the neurodegenerative diseases [47]. The abnormal pathologic proteins include alpha-synuclein, tau, beta-amyloid, and prion [48]. In Parkinson's [49] and Huntington's diseases [50], these proteins are accumulated in the cytosol. Aggregation of these intracellular toxic proteins in the cell nucleus causes spinocerebellar ataxia type 1 [51]. Here comes the role of autophagy. Autophagy is the best mechanism that clear the cell of toxic proteins. Activation of autophagy through genetic signaling (autophagy-related genes, ATG) would increase the scavenging mechanism for the toxic proteins preventing their aggregation inside the cell. Therefore, their damaging effect is eliminated. Defective autophagy or failure of maturation of the autophagy process by any factor would augment the aggregation of the mutant proteins leading to disease development [48].

That is why autophagy is designated as a guardian against neurodegenerative diseases.

It has been found that pharmacological stimulation of autophagy will decrease the levels of soluble as well as aggregated mutant proteins in most of the previously mentioned neurodegenerative diseases. These researches are supported by the animal models of neurodegenerative diseases. In line with this process, reduction of the efficacy of ATG genes (knockdown) or rendering the genes inoperative (knockout) will lead to the formation of aggregate-prone proteins with their toxic impact over the cells [52]. It has been claimed that the neuro protection medicated by the autophagy is the result of the reduction of the amount of mutant toxic proteins would be attributed to antiapoptotic effects [46].

Apart from defective autophagy, the capacity of autophagy may be exceeded to a point beyond which the autophagy cannot scavenge the excessive amount of toxic mutant proteins anymore. Sequestration of autophagy proteins in the aggregates formed by the abnormal proteins may contribute to defective autophagy auto phagosome generation. The net result is the accumulation of the abnormal toxic proteins inside the cell. Auto phagosome-generation defect can also occur as a result of the aging of autophagy proteins causing this useful protein to decline from the cell. Other autophagy proteins are as-of-yet undefined may contribute to the malfunction of autophagy resulting in accumulation of the harmful proteins [48], [53].

The available data is considered the bases for the initiation of clinical trials using agents that stimulate autophagy. These agents have shown encouraging results in minimizing the neurotoxicity of the aggregate-prone proteins. Rapamycin analogs, for example, are proved to give promising results in managing the neurodegenerative disorders. These agents are primarily designated for guarding against organ transplant rejection and preventing restenosis after coronary angioplasty [54]. Also, lithium chloride, a bipolar disorder therapy, gives promising results in activating autophagy and clearing the cell off the proteins aggregates [55]. It is interesting to know that these agents have potentiality in preventing aging process by preventing the decline in autophagy protein expression in the nervous system and removal of lysosomes by autophagy; these processes are involved in the aging process [3].

Liver disease

It has been believed that autophagy in the liver can play a dual effect. On one hand, autophagy can protect the liver cells from cancer and on the other autophagy can support tumor cell survival or fibrosis formation. Liver cells protection by autophagy is represented by removing damaged organelles, enhancing protein breakdown, and promoting cell differentiation. Moreover, hepatic autophagy can induce cell death of the malignant cells as well. However, autophagy can help cancer growth through recycling of nutrients and production of energy [56]. This dual effect of hepatic autophagy has its implications on the therapeutic strategy of anticancer treatment. The therapeutic strategy should concern the induction of autophagy pathway that suppresses cancer attributes and inhibiting autophagy pathway that encourages cancer development [57].

Autophagy has an important role in protecting the liver from the accumulation of large fat droplets rich in triglycerides inside the cells (steatosis). Steatosis occurs in alcoholic patients leading to various forms of liver toxicity. Alcoholism induces steatosis by compromising the function of autophagy [58]. Recent studies prove that pharmacological up-regulation of autophagy function contributes to the prevention of steatosis and guards the liver cells against the toxic effect of fat accumulation [59], [60]. Up-regulation of autophagy removes the damaged mitochondria as well as the accumulated fat droplets.

Source [60]. Therefore, the up-regulation of autophagy is the primary treatment against steatosis.

Autophagy acts through a cell-intrinsic mechanism to mediate inhibition of new cancer formation (carcinogenesis). [61]. The degrading power of autophagy disrupts the genomic material needed for the development of hepatocellular cancer (HCC) in patients with virus C infection HCV [62]. Defective autophagy is strongly associated with poor outcome of HCC.

It has been noticed that intact autophagy enhances virus C replication in the liver. Autophagy is exploited by virus C to assemble infectious virus particles (virions). Virus C utilizes the autophagy proteins (i.e. Beclin-1, Atg4b, and others) for the translation of the viral RNA genome and the production of the virions [63].

Autophagy exerts a quality control of proteins through the disposition of aggregate-prone proteins in the basal liver cells similar to that in the brain cells (neurons). The quality control of protein is supposed to be important in the development of $\alpha 1$-antitrypsin deficiency. It is a genetic liver disease characterized by features of chronic inflammation and cancer formation (carcinogenesis) [64]. Liver cells with $\alpha 1$-antitrypsin deficiency exhibit a mutation in $\alpha 1$-

antitrypsin Z gene point. The resulting mutation leads to the generation of proteins with abnormal folding structure and tendency to form aggregates within the endoplasmic reticulum (ER) of the liver cell. Unlike the normally generated $\alpha 1$-antitrypsin, the mutant $\alpha 1$-antitrypsin Z is cleared off the liver cells mainly by the autophagy. Therefore, defective autophagy results in decreased $\alpha 1$-antitrypsin Z degradation and increase of cytoplasmic aggregates. The transgenic expression of $\alpha 1$-antitrypsin Z triggers the function of autophagy in vivo studies [65] . It has been suggested that such aggregates cause sequestration of autophagy proteins resulting in a reduction of the cytoprotective action and elimination of tumor suppressor effect of autophagy [66].

Muscle disease

The effect of autophagy in muscle degenerative disease is similar to what has been discussed for neurodegenerative diseases. For example, Danon disease is a genetic myopathic disease linked to chromosome X. Danon disease affects mainly the heart, muscles, and the brain. It is characterized by lysosomal and glycogen storage abnormality [67]. Danon disease shows a mutation in the lysosome protein designated as LAMP-2. The defective mutant protein is associated with a tremendous increase in auto phagosomes in muscle cells due to the failure to fuse with lysosomes [68]. Similar results can be reached by applying pharmacological inhibition on the process of auto phagosomes fusion with lysosomes [69].

Moreover, the defective lysosomal function can be pathogenic due to the accumulation of graded material, for example, in Pompe disease. Mutation in the GAA gene in Pompe disease causes a deficiency in α-glucosidase enzyme. This enzyme is responsible for glycogen breakdown to glucose by lysosomes. This leads to an accumulation of glycogen in auto phagosomes resulting in cell damage [70]. This is a good example of how excessive accumulation of graded material by itself could be harmful to the cell. The accumulated debris causes "traffic jam" that prevents the beneficial effect of replacement therapy. Autophagy needs to be suppressed to allow for replacement therapy [71]

Cancer

Autophagy represents a double-edged sword in facing the tumor cells. Under certain contexts in the cell, excessive stimulation of cancer cell autophagy may be pro-death rather than pro-survival for tumor cells. This tragedy fate occurs in the cell where apoptosis (programmed cell death) is defective. The understanding of the role of autophagy in cancer etiology and development is crucial in the development of pharmacotherapy for cancer.

The pro-death role of autophagy for tumor generation is represented by removal of the aged organelles, protection of the genome, and turnover of proteins. Therefore, the biological generation of cell nutrients is maintained, and the tumor cell nutrients are disposed of. The vitality of the normal cell is, likewise, preserved and the precancerous processes are either reversed to protect the cell from turning into frank malignancy or the cells are destroyed (hence, pre-death). Consequently, homeostasis is settled. Several findings have proved the undenied role of autophagy in the management of cancer. Cells with defective autophagy have shown to be related to tumor generation. Moreover, cells with Beclin 1 gene defect is lacking Beclin 1 protein that is important for the functionality of autophagy. This defect leads to the development of several types of cancers such as breast and ovarian cancer in females, prostate cancer in males. In these types of cancer, Beclin 1 defect was found in 40-75% [72].

The pro-survival pathway comes in favor of tumor cell development and progression. Under certain contexts, autophagy confers stress tolerance for tumor cells allowing them to survive and progress. Stress in tumor cells is related to the increased demand for metabolites due to the rapid replication of the tumor cells. These stressful conditions trigger autophagy for the benefit of cancer cell survival. Also, lack of oxygen (hypoxia) in the tumor environment, due to the rapid proliferation of tumor cells, is considered a stressful condition as well. Therefore, autophagy is triggered to enable the cell to stand the stress. This mechanism comes to the benefit of the tumor cell. The activation of autophagy under such stressful conditions not only plays a role in the vitality of the tumor cells but act as a pathway that is resistance to treatment as well.

The pro-survival pathway, therefore, is a new target for cancer therapy. Several studies have proved that the suppression of the pro-survival pathway of autophagy is greatly beneficial in killing the tumor cells [73]. When the prosurvival autophagy is suppressed either by genetic or pharmacological means, cell death is triggered leading to the elimination of tumor cells successfully. The suppression of autophagy leads to activation of apoptosis that suppress tumor cell growth and development [74]. The clinical studies have proved that this strategy gives more successful results than relying on conventional chemotherapy alone [75].

In clinical trials, inhibition of autophagy makes the cells sensitive to medications. That is to say, the tumor cell becomes more respondent to treatment. This was proved successful in leukemia and colon cancer where apoptosis is defective [76]. Cetuximab is an antibody that docks on the receptors for the growth factor of the epidermis. This antibody is used as a medication for colon cancer treatment. The effect of cetuximab is mediated by inhibition of the pro-survival pathway of autophagy. The net result is activation of the programmed cell death (apoptosis) and termination of cancer cells [77]. Several other pharmacological agents are under trial acting on inhibiting autophagy [78].

Chapter 4:
Autophagy and Aging

Introduction

It has been observed that many biological changes are affected by aging. Biologically, aging is a group of progressive, yet predictable changes. These changes will lead to increased susceptibility to disease. This means that the person becomes more prone to be afflicted by certain diseases than before- a young age. There are many factors affect the aging process such as the genetic makeup of the person and the environmental factors. The genetic factors constitute around 25% of the variation in longevity while the environmental factors account for 50% [79].

What does really happen in our body when we are aging? The physiological process in our body is subject to a rhythmic pattern. The circadian pattern, for example, of body temperature, secretion of cortisol, and sleep pattern are all impacted by the advance in age. Hormones are secreted in a pulsatile form such as gonadotropins in females (fertility hormone), growth hormone (for cell growth and maturation), thyrotropin (stimulate the thyroid gland for facilitating energy production), melatonin (responsible for skin coloration), and adrenocorticotropin hormone (for facing stress). With the advance of age, this pulsatile form is lost. Moreover, our physiologic reserves are depleted. The balance between the formation of new material and the consumption of these materials is called homeostasis. When the balance between synthesis and consumption is disrupted, the body suffers "Homeostenosis." This term was designated by Walter Cannon in 1940 [80], [81]. Homeostenosis renders the body susceptible to diseases that occur mostly when we advance in age.

Autophagy and quality control

We recall that autophagy is considered as an evolutionary pathway that is present in most organisms from years that have only one cell to flies, rats, and mammals with many cells (multicellular organisms. Autophagy function is to maintain protein and organelle *quality control* in the cell. The quality control is achieved by elimination of unfolded or altered proteins and aged organelles. Also, the so-called aged structures are removed from the cell by the autophagy process. The resulting outcome is amino acids and fatty acids that are engaged once more in the biosynthesis of proteins and organelles that are not only new but beneficial to the survival of the cell.

In essence, autophagy is the guard against cell disruption is decay or tumor development. A large body of evidence supports that defective autophagy is associated with the development of age-related diseases such as neurodegenerative diseases [44], [48] and cancer [28]. Moreover, mounting evidence suggests that in aging organisms, the autophagy influence exerted on multiple human metabolic pathophysiological processes for the survival and protection of the cell has become insufficient- the principle of homeostenosis [53] . This insufficiency of the autophagy functions leads to age-related metabolic diseases such as diabetes millets , morbid obesity [83], non-alcoholic steatohepatitis (accumulation of fat in the liver in non-alcoholic persons) [84], and atherosclerosis (artery disease with deposition of fatty plaques on the walls) [85].

Aging Process

Decreased or inhibited autophagy in advance of age has been found in tremendously in a variety of "aging" systems. The early studies of autophagy and aging identified the role of autophagy genes in model organisms. A model organism is a non-human species e.g. yeast, fly, or rat that is submitted to experimentation to provide us with insight into how our body works. This technique is resorted to when to research a human disease or new therapies when human experimentation is impractical or unethical. A model organism such as yeast (Saccharomyces cerevisiae), nematode (Caenorhabditis elegans), and fruit fly (Drosophila melanogaster) showed reduced lifespan in mutants defective in the expression of genes designated as Atg1 and Atg8 [86]. The gene deletion technique was helpful to underscore the crucial effect of the autophagy genes (Atg) in quality control, generations of cell organelles, and cell differentiation. However, deletion of Atg7 and Atg8 genes (knockout) in young mice does not show fatality. Rather, age-related disorders are evolved similar to that developed in advanced age such as accumulation of intracellular aggregation with neurodegeneration [87], accumulation of lysosomes filled with pigment lipofuscin [88], and decreased muscle mass as observed in sarcopenia (a disease of loss of muscle bulk and function with aging) [89].

These studies cast light on the determining role of autophagy quality control in the aging process. As the autophagy quality control is waning off, several toxic materials accumulate extensively over time contributing to the age-related pathology. The age-related pathology associated with waning off the quality control includes reduced muscle mass, neurodegeneration, heart disorders, accumulation of lipid of the arterial wall (atherogenesis) and insulin insensitivity.

The second factor that would come into play in determining tissue loss with age is tissue differentiation. Cell differentiation is a process by which a cell changes from one type to another which is usually more specialized in function. Recent studies on depletion of Atg7 in adulthood life showed that cells deficient in Atg7 gene causes brown adipose tissue to lose specialization and function i.e. dedifferentiation. As a result, lipid accumulation is promoted [85]. Therefore, it is likely that autophagy waning off with age contribute to loss of muscle or brown fat cell specialization resulting in loss of their functional characteristics. The net result is the disruption of tissue function.

Defective genome maintenance is the third-tier undermining cell function caused by loss of autophagy with age. Recent studies have identified the significant role of autophagy genes products in guarding against genomic destruction and promoting genomic repair [90], [91]. Autophagy acts as a scavenging process for removal of oxidative stress condition and cumulative toxic insults that can damage the DNA genome and accelerate either cell death or cancer development. More studies are needed to elucidate the role of autophagy in guarding the cell genome and prevent genome damage.

The question that arises now is why autophagy function decline with age. The answer is not straightforward. The autophagy and aging are two complex processes with many factors operating for them. It has been suggested that down-regulation of Atg5 and Atg7 gene transcription that has been detected in human brain cells are associated with normal aging [92]. Moreover, it has been noticed that the degrading enzymes (proteolytic enzymes) have been decreased with age in model organisms [93]. It has been suggested that abnormal regulation of autophagy is secondary to the aberration of hormonal responses to starvation and defective metabolism. For examples, with the advance of age, the stimulatory effect of glucagon on autophagy is fading while the inhibitory effect of insulin remains intact [93], [94]. The result is down-regulation of autophagy with age and the occurrence of the related consequences ending with the death of the organism.

Chapter 5:
Autophagy and obesity

Introduction

Lipids (fats) are the fuel for cell energy. They are the main components that provide the cells with a tremendous amount of energy. The cells utilize the energy produced by fat metabolism to perform the specified functions. The second most important function of lipid is the formation of the cell membrane and the membranes of the other biological structures within the cell. Lysosomes play an essential role in the recycling process of lipids. First, lipids are delivered to lysosomes by autophagy for their degradation. Then, lysosomes that contain hydrolytic enzymes degrade lipids to the basic components- fatty acids. Finally, the products of lipid degradation (catabolites) are, then, redistributed to every cell parts to underpin the basic cellular function [84]. There has been a dual relationship between lysosomes and lipids. Lysosomes, on one hand, regulate lipid metabolism inside the cell. On the other hand, lipids promote the functions of lysosomes as well as autophagy.

The principle of autophagy has been applied to reduce the weight of obese persons and to prevent the development of related diseases. For instance, during the periods of fasting, autophagy is triggered by fast stress. The activated autophagy acts to remove the fat droplets from inside of the cells and use the degeneration products for energy production. Intermittent fasting without supplying the body with fat will force the cells to use the stored fat as a fuel or a building block. The net result is the consumption of body fat and loss of weight.

Role of Autophagy in Fat Metabolism

Fat (lipid) metabolism has garnered the attention of scientific research due to the potential implications in obesity and the related syndromes [95]. Several studies conducted on the cultured hepatocytes showed that fat droplets are selectively seized in auto phagosomes and delivered to lysosomes. There is an enzyme system called lysosomal acid lipases that is responsible for the degradation of fat droplets inside the lysosomes. This process is called "lipophagy." It is a distinct mechanism from the conventional fat metabolism pathway [96].

There is an intricate relationship between obesity and autophagy. In essence, autophagy plays a critical role in the development and progress of obesity and related pathology. Obesity is associated with various pathological features including accumulation of fat droplets, protein aggregates, and non-functioning mitochondria. These are supposed to be substrates for autophagy. Therefore, it has been presumed that the abrogation of autophagy is associated with obesity-related pathology in the cells of multiple tissue systems [83]. This hypothesis has been suggested by the finding that ablation of genetic autophagy in liver cells leads to the observation of pathological features resembling that in non-alcoholic steatohepatitis. These features are directly related to autophagy including the formation of protein inclusion, accumulation of fat droplets, and liver cell injury [97].

It has been observed that autophagy up regulation occurs prior to obesity-related morbidity. The explanation is that autophagy guard against accumulation fat droplets within the cell in case of morbid obesity. However, the final outcome varies according to certain circumstances. For example, in type 2 diabetic patients with insulin resistance (unresponsiveness of the cell to insulin given to the patient), autophagy upregulation has been demonstrated. Together with the simultaneous increase of fat droplets, the degradation products, free fatty acids, are excessively released favoring cellular toxicity. This notion opens the door for the creation of pharmacological agents that would either block or downregulate autophagy to a normal level with promising results [98].

Chapter 6:
Our Feeding Habit

Our Eating Habits

The recent discovery of autophagy and its effect on health, aging, and disease highlighted the need to review our eating habits. Humans and other animals feed to supply their bodies with energy and the necessary elements for maintaining life. Hunger is the psycho-physiological process that alarms humans about the need to fuel. Hunger is one process that keeps humans' life intact. However, we don't usually eat because we are hungry. We usually eat out of habit rather than out of hunger.

Food and advertisement are everywhere around us. The media, websites, and streets have a tempting advertisement for food of various kinds. This temptation makes us carve for food and shape up our eating habit to what is called the "Western eating habits." Fast food is everywhere and at our fingertips-"home delivery."

Overweight and obesity

The world health organization admitted that overweight is an epidemic disease affecting 39% of people above the age of 18. This means that 1.9B person is overweight worldwide. The worst is that 41M children under the age of 5 are obese [99].

The difference between overweight and obesity is calculated by the body mass index (BMI). BMI is your weight in kilograms (Kg) divided by the square of your height in meters (m^2). When your BMI lies somewhere between 25 and 30 you are overweight. Obese people have their BMI exceeding 30. BMI is a good estimate of obesity in men and women and for adults and children. The relationship between obesity and heart disease and stroke has been established. Heart disease has been on the top list of the leading causes of death [100]. Muscle diseases and some types of cancer (breast, uterus, ovaries, prostate, liver) are strongly associated with obesity [100].

Time to change

Now, it is time to think about changing our eating habits. Three meals a day with three snacks or more should be reconsidered. For losing weight, changing the pattern of eating is equally important to change the type of food. Autophagy science tells us that the time of eating is of utmost importance in weight loss. Also, the time interval between meals is of utmost importance in reducing weight, keeping our skin young, and beating disease of old age. The spacing between meals is known as the "fasting periods."

When we space between meals, we create a time of nutrition deprivation. At this time of deprivation, the cell is stressed leading to activation of autophagy. It has been documented that promoting autophagy is effective in weight loss. When time spacing between food reaches 16hrs, autophagy is found to be activated. This is called "intermittent fasting."

Fasting

Abstinence of food or drink for a specific period of time is called *fasting*. We need to know two types of fasting: the dry fasting which is abstinence of all food and drink for a d defined period of the day; water fasting that refers to abstinence from all food and fluids except water.

<u>Ancient traditions</u>

Fast is observed by religious traditions namely Islam, Christianity, and Judaism. Fasting includes all or most of the food and drink for a variable period of time of the day.

Islam and Judaism observe fasting for most of the day that is considered close to the modern intermittent fasting. Other faith and "religions" observed fasting as well such as Buddhism, Hinduism, Sikhism, and Taoism. The common thing in the ancient fasting tradition is the concern about health and beating disease.

At that time, it was a matter of intuition or trial and error. Modern science has come to prove that the ancient tradition was right. Fasting, now, is a recommended pattern of eating for health and beating disease on solid scientific bases. You don't need to follow any tradition to fast. You can just make up your mind and start fasting for your health and beating disease. It is our modern twenty-one-century tradition.

Patterns of modern fasting

It is the time of abstinence from food that autophagy is activated and perform the regeneration process. There are different proposed types of fasting. The first approach is fasting for 24hrs twice a week. It is harsh and non-applicable. The second approach is fasting for 16hrs and 8hrs "feeding period" every day. The third approach suggests one large meal a day and fasting the rest of the day. The last approach is subject to multiple snacks during the fasting period. The fourth approach is an alternate day approach. The person eats diet low in calories in one day and the second day is free. This pattern will be alternating every second day.

The main issue in the intermittent fasting approach is to allow the body to feel stressed and deficient of nutrients. Exerting stress over the body will enforce the cells to initiate the autophagy process. Intermittent fasting and low-calorie diets work well for weight loss. Both mechanisms act together to stimulate autophagy in our cell bodies. It has been found that short periods of fasting activates autophagy in the brain cells. The implications of autophagy in beating the development of neurodegenerative diseases such as Parkinson's disease and Alzheimer's disease [86] as well as guarding against mood and emotions disorders such as depression and anxiety [101].

Another type of autophagy diet approach is *ketosis*. Ketosis promotes autophagy in the brain. The implications of ketosis diet sound great in protecting our brain cells in many aspects [102]. In the following chapter, we will discuss ketosis in detail.

Autophagy might suites you or not

One may be skeptical of applying new regimen for diet. Some public regimens are proved non-scientific and depend on mere personal experience. Some regimens are proved non-effective or even harmful. Autophagy, on the contrary, carries growing scientific support. Recent researches provide strong evidence-based ground for the implementation of autophagy and hence, intermittent fasting, for weight loss regimens, skin care, disease protection, to name a few.

Intermittent fasting is not harmful to you. The most important point in the diet is safety and efficacy. Many people do not cope with diet restriction for days or months. They may revert to their usual dietary habits once the restriction is relived. Diet should keep you in a good mood either mentally or physically. Intermittent fasting has all that you are looking for.

Some people are not fit for dropping out breakfast. They feel drown out of energy. They feel headache, agitated, and nervous. They may lose concentration that would have serious implication on their work performance or academic attention. So, dropping out of breakfast is not recommended for them.

Protein recipes in breakfast, however, would make them feel full and satiate. Protein can be consumed by the body as a source of energy. Therefore, they will not feel confused and not-concentrated. It is the response of your body, your brain that would choose what is good for you, what suits you best.

Chapter 7:
Ketones Impact on Human performance

What are ketones?

Ketones are simple compounds made of carbon, hydrogen, and oxygen. They are the result of fat degradation in the body and are a rich source of energy as well. The process that utilizes ketones is called ketosis. Three different, yet chemically related, ketones are identified. They are acetoacetate, beta-hydroxybutyrate, and acetone. The three ketones, also called ketone bodies, dissolves in water easily i.e. water-soluble compounds.

Ketones are produced in the liver, muscle, and brain cells as well as mitochondria-rich cells in our body under stressful conditions. Our body resorts to the utilization of ketones as an alternative source of energy to glucose in stressful conditions such as fasting, low carbs intake, intense exercise, alcoholism, and starvation. Unlike other cells in the body, the liver cells have the necessary machinery to generate glucose out of ketones. The process of generating glucose from sources other than carbs is called gluconeogenesis.

Gluconeogenesis is activated in the liver cells under the time of stress. During fasting (usually 72 hours) or low carbs, diet insulin level decreases and glucagon and corticosteroid hormones are elevated. The hormonal response to fasting initiates the gluconeogenesis process to compensate for the lack of glucose in the blood. Moreover, muscles and brain cells, among other cells, shifts from using glucose as an energy source to using ketones instead.

The heart can utilize fatty acids under normal conditions. Under stressful conditions when ketones increase in the blood, the heart can effectively utilize ketones for energy and maintain functions.

Brain cell uses glucose preferentially. The brain cell prefers to use fatty acids and ketones to generate the cell membrane rather than the production of energy. In cases of fasting or starvation, the brain uses glucose obligatorily. After 3 days under adverse conditions, the brain starts to get 25% of its energy out of ketone bodies [103]. After 24 days of fasting or low-carb diet, ketones replace glucose for energy production [104]. Ketones make up to two-thirds of fuel used by the brain cells. The speculation that the brain can survive with ketones only cannot be proved due to ethical restrictions. It is worth mentioning that ketones produced from omega-3 fatty acids may exert a deleterious effect on the cognitive function of aged persons [105].

Ketones and performance

Nutritional strategies target human performance to a great extent. Anecdotally, ketone supplements would induce ketosis fast without the need for diet restriction. In 1983, the principle of ketones supplements as performance enhancer was first introduced. The main idea is that chronic ketosis without restriction of caloric intake will preserve glycogen in the body and conserve carbohydrate consumption that is lacking under stressful conditions [106]. It is expected that such an approach would reserve adequate exercise capacity. The research studies about the efficacy of ketones diet in promoting performance is conflicting. The conflicting results of the studies underlie the complexity of ketosis as a performance enhancer.

The Definition of Health

Health has been defined by the Constitution of the World Health Organization, April 7, 1948, as " a state of complete physical, mental, and social wellbeing, and not merely the absence of disease or infirmity"[107].

Today, three concepts of the definition of health occupy our minds. The first concept is simply the absence of disease or impairment. However, chronically ill patients such as those with controlled hypertension or well-adjusted diabetes can do well in their life with the little negative impact of the disease for a long period of time.

The second concept is that health is a state that enables the person to cope with all daily life requirements adequately. Although this concept includes the absence of disease, it also includes those who are chronically ill and stable.

The third concept is a state of equilibrium that is established between the person and himself and between the person the surrounding environment [108]. This concept would consider hypertensive patients healthy when they achieve balance with the environment that makes them get the most out of their life despite being designated by professionals as ill [109].

In 1943, the French physician, Georges Canguilhem, opposed the previous notion about health. Canguilhem rejected that health is either normal or abnormal. From his point of view, health cannot be defined by statistical procedures or mechanistically. On the contrary, according to Canguilhem, health is not a fixed entity, rather, it is the ability of the person to adapt to the surrounding environment considering the person's circumstances. This concept of Canguilhem makes health a definition by you and me not by the physician. It is you and I who determine if we adapt will with the environment or not. The mere role of the physician is to help us to adapt to the environment according to the current condition. This notion heralded the emergence of what is called "personalized medicine" [108].

Ketones and Brain Diseases

The accumulating body of evidence showed that ketones play an important role in minimizing the neurodegenerative brain diseases. Alzheimer's disease, for example, can be challenged by ketones. However, the basis of the effect of ketone diet on the neurodegenerative diseases is not fully understood.

It has been suggested that autophagy may mediate the action of ketone diet on the brain cells. Upregulation of neuronal autophagy is proved to share in the neuroprotective efforts of ketones to guard the brain against degenerative disease. Autophagy destroys damaged mitochondria to prevent superoxide excessive production and free radicals. Activated autophagy eliminates protein aggregates that modulate the neurodegenerative disease.

Agents that can permeate the brain barrier such as metformin and berberine have a potential effect in enhancing ketones formation and boosting autophagy.

People have the choice to either follow the ketogenic diet or follow an alternative strategy when a ketogenic diet regimen is intolerable. The alternative regimen include eating a diet rich in medium-chain triglycerides, coconut oil, and intermittent ketogenic diet rather than a continuous diet. Moreover, food supplements that enhance ketogenesis in the liver cells. Other suggested strategy is having supplements that enhance ketogenesis in the liver cells such as carnitine and hydroxy-citrate. The latter regimen should be combined with a fasting program or abstinence from carbs diet [110].

The ketogenic diet regiment will be discussed in the following chapters. In the next section, we are discussing the influence of ketosis on the course of neurovegetative diseases such as Alzheimer's disease and Parkinson's disease.

<u>Ketones challenge Alzheimer's disease</u>

The brain cells of patients suffering from Alzheimer's disease cannot get the benefit of glucose for energy production. Most cortical areas in the brain of afflicted persons show decreased metabolism and energy production. Deficient metabolism is attributed to the cognitive symptoms of Alzheimer's disease.

The brain cells have reduced insulin receptors in certain regions of the cortex. This means that insulin will not be able to dock on the cell wall of the brain cells and sends signals to start glucose utilization. This situation resembles insulin resistance in diabetic patients type 2. Dr. de la Monte and colleagues pointed out that Alzheimer's disease as a neuroendocrine disease is similar to type 2 diabetes in the fact that the cells cannot utilize glucose properly due to lack of insulin signals. Unlike the brain cells, the muscle cells, for example, can use fat stores to produce energy. He designated Alzheimer's disease like diabetes type 3 for this reason [111].

When the brain cells cannot utilize glucose, it accumulates in the brain causing oxidative stress and damage to the cells. Also, the brain cells utilize glucose in obligation to get the energy they need. Without energy, the cells starve and finally die.

Ketones, otherwise, are an alternative source for fuel and energy in this case. When you adjust your diet to be low in carbs, your body shifts to ketones for the production of energy. This will help to treat the disease. Numerous recent studies support this notion to a great extent. Ketones are shown to bypass the inability to use glucose for energy [112], block amyloid formation (a plaque accumulating in the Alzheimer's disease) [113], improvement of brain cognitive function [114]in the afflicted persons.

In conclusion, a diet that induces ketones is a promising approach in managing patients with neurodegenerative diseases including Alzheimer's.

Ketones and seizures

Seizures are another brain disorder that can benefit from a ketone diet. Seizures are abrupt, out of control electrical disturbance in the brain cells. The brain cells at a certain locus fire automatically and out of control. Seizures are the result of the loss of balance between the excitatory and inhibitory impulses in the brain. The electrical imbalance causes chemical changes leading to surges in electrical activity and hence, seizures.

In fact, seizures are not a disease, rather, it is a symptom of a disease. When someone has a specific brain disorder, they are liable to have seizures.

Seizures are noticed following brain stroke, head injury, and brain infection e.g. meningitis.

The outcome of seizures depends on the site of the brain with increased cell firing. Seizures can affect the behavior, movement, or feeling of the afflicted persons. Epilepsy is a disease that is diagnosed when two or more seizures episodes occur with a tendency for recurrence.

Ketone bodies are shown to have anti-seizure properties. Beta-hydroxybutyrate is found to hit several target receptors (docking sites) on immune cells [115]. However, when it comes to diet therapy, it is difficult to specify one single mechanism of action. Diet therapy renders a battery of biochemical, molecular, and cellular changes. Beta-hydroxybutyrate is one substrate of many in the ketonic diet that can affect brain hyperexcitable state and hypersynchrony.

In 1920, a diet low in carbs and high in fat was developed by a healer to help children with epileptic fits [116]. Although the diet content was anecdotal, the children were improved to some extent. The recent development of anti-epileptic medications rendered that formula unfavorable by the scientific community. That formula, now called a ketogenetic diet, was creating a state similar to carbs starvation.

Recently, the ketogenic diet attracted the attention of researchers and clinicians for its undenied effect on epilepsy. However, it is resorted to in resistant cases and some odd forms of epilepsy. We wonder if the comeback of the ketogenic diet should be welcomed or damped. The ongoing studies should answer this query.

There is growing evidence that ketone bodies function exceeds the role of cellular fuel agents. Ketone bodies are found to have strong biochemical, cellular, and epigenetic changes. These changes are so powerful that they can decrease the excitability of the complex brain networks [117]. The exceeded function of ketone bodies is mediated via both inhibitory and excitatory neurotransmission. Moreover, ketone bodies target mitochondria affecting the respiratory chain [118].

The anti-epileptic effect can be directly on the excited cells, however, there is no valid evidence yet. However, clinical trials on animal models proved that ketone diet with low-carbs and high-fat content can reduce the flare of the epileptic episodes. These results are so promising for future therapeutic implications of ketonic diet [117].

Parkinson's disease and ketogenic diet

Parkinson's disease is a degenerative disorder of the brain cells affecting the motor system. The disease is associated with dementia and depression as well. The afflicted person suffers from shaking, rigid muscles, slow movement, and difficulty in speech. Later, the advance of the disease is related to dementia, depression, and anxiety.

The exact cause of the disease is not clear. It is believed to be an interplay between genetic and environmental factors. Cell death in the substantia nigra (black substance) in the midbrain could be the main reason for motor dysfunction. These show a low level of dopamine transmitter. Moreover, abnormal protein aggregate are shown called Lewy bodies [119].

To date, recent research discovered several genes that are directly related to the inherited familial form of Parkinson's disease. The mutations on these genes are directly associated with mitochondria dysfunction. The most recent studies supported the role of these genes in controlling the function of mitochondria. Moreover, new genes have been identified with direct relation to mitochondrial function and dysfunction. The new discoveries underpin the important role of mitochondrial function in the development of Parkinson's disease.

The mitochondrial abnormalities occur earlier than dopamine deficiency [120].

The ketogenic diet has been proved to improve the motor and non-motor symptoms in patients with Parkinson's disease. The effect of the ketogenic diet exceeds that of a high-fat diet [121]. However, studies have conflicting results as regards the ratio of fat-to-carbs in the diet. Matthew Phillips, MSc, Waikato Hospital, Hamilton, New Zealand, and colleagues have conducted a pilot study to compare the effect of a ketogenic diet with a diet that contains low fat. The sample involved patients with Parkinson's disease in a hospital. Dr. Phillips described the diet plan as "simple, affordable, and palatable." The result of Dr. Phillips research showed great improvement in non-motor symptoms such as urinary problems, pain, fatigue, daytime sleeping, and cognitive dysfunction. "…, notably, represent some of the more disabling, less levodopa-responsive nonmotor symptoms in Parkinson's." [122].

One modality suggested for the beneficial effect of ketogenic diet in patients with Parkinson's disease is the promising effect on mitochondria. Studies conducted on animal models proved that ketones are of great importance in restoring the respiratory function of mitochondria.

On such studies showed that giving mice a ketone body, d-beta-hydroxybutyrate confers partial protection against the deleterious effect of brain cell damage at the regions where dopamine is produced. The end result is the improvement of mitochondrial respiration with the production of ATP (adenosine triphosphate- the fuel of the cell) [123].

Another study on rat models found that the ketogenic diet enhances brain metabolism. The main impact of the ketogenic diet was enforcing mitochondria to perform better under low-glucose conditions. The study suggests that the anticonvulsant mechanism of the ketogenic diet involves biogenesis of mitochondria boosting alternative energy stores [124]. That is to say, mitochondria, the powerhouse of the cell, would increase in number, therefore, an enhancement in energy production is expected.

Moreover, rat model provided us with the evidence that ketogenic diet help guards against free radicals' production by mitochondria. Therefore, the oxidative stress is reduced protecting the cells from the harmful effect of the free radicals. Ketogenic diet boosts glutathione generation with elevating the ability of mitochondrial antioxidant pathways. This mechanism protects mtDNA genome from damage by oxidation [125]. This effect is also beneficial in reducing seizures in epileptic patients [125].

Ketogenic diet and metabolism

Metabolism is a set of chemical reactions inside the cell for turning food into energy, generation of building blocks for proteins, fats, and nucleic acid, and get rid of waste byproducts.

Ketones are known to affect metabolism in different ways. Ketones reduce insulin release and replace glucose as a fuel source. Ketones suppress appetite enforcing weight loss without suffering hunger. Finally, ketones reduce cholesterol level in blood including triglycerides and LDL. The direct effect of low cholesterol has decreased the risk of heart stroke and angina (chest pain of cardiac origin).

Ketogenic diet and insulin level

Insulin is a protein hormone released from the Langerhans' islets in the Pancreas. Insulin docs on the cell wall (insulin receptor) to send signals to the cell to utilize glucose for energy. Insulin is released from Langerhans' islets in response to blood glucose surge. This surge occurs immediately after meals rich in carbs.

High ketone diet decreases glucose blood level and hence, the insulin level decreases accordingly.

During prolonged fasting, the body shifts to fatty acids as an alternative source of energy. Fatty acids yield ketone bodies that block glucose release and consequently, insulin release will be inhibited.

When insulin increases during fasting hours (hyperinsulinemia) are linked with chronic diseases. Moreover, high fasting insulin is linked to cancer as well. Recent studies show that diabetes type 2 is associated with an increased incidence of mortality from cancer. The progression of cancer in type 2 diabetes as well as in obesity is contributed partially to high blood glucose level, high fasting insulin (hyperinsulinemia), insulin-like growth factor 1, abnormal lipids (dyslipidemia) and gut microbiome as a short list [126]. The deleterious effect of high fasting insulin in raising the risk of cancer is proved to be independent of diabetes and obesity [127]. Therefore, reducing insulin level is expected to reduce the risk of cancer.

Long before the onset of diabetes, insulin resistance may develop with increased fasting insulin level. There have been speculations that high insulin level under such circumstances is causally linked to vessel diseases. This leads to the development of atherosclerosis (accumulation of lipid plagues on the wall of the blood vessels). It is obvious that the developed atherosclerosis has its implications in hypertension, coronary stroke (angina) and cerebral stroke [128].

Ketones are postulated to have therapeutic implications in patients with insulin resistance and high insulin level. The suggested mechanism is probably mediated by alteration of the mitochondrial respiratory pathway [129].

Insulin is needed for glucose burn. Fat can be burned without the need for glucose. Therefore, supplying the body with ketones or ketogenic diet with high-fat, low-carbs will force the body to shift away from glucose as a fuel and start utilizing fat for fuel. This is exactly what we are apt to. The net result is a reduction of insulin level with decreased risk of disease mortality. So, the recommended diet is high fat, moderate protein, and low carbs.

Ketogenic diet and appetite

Hunger and appetite are controlled by the interplay of two hormones in our body. They are called leptin and ghrelin hormones. Leptin hormone is generated by fat cells. Leptin function is to decrease appetite. It let us feel satiated. It has been found that leptin is normally low in thin persons and quite high in fat persons. However, this is not always the case. Fat people are not affected by leptin hormone. It seems that leptin works no more. This is called *resistance.* The body of the obese persons resist the action of leptin hormone and respond no more to its action. That is why obese (fat) persons usually feel hungry and abstinence of food is a big problem for them.

On the other hand, ghrelin hormone increases appetite. Ghrelin makes you feel hungry and carving for food. It is secreted mainly in our stomachs. When ghrelin is released, it sends signals to our brain to feel hungry. Then, the hormone decreases three hours after meals. Normally, ghrelin hormone increases when the person is lean and decreases when the person is obese.

Ghrelin hormone is released when the stomach is empty. Empty stomach means a need for food. So, the ghrelin cell in the wall of the stomach starts secreting the hormone. On the other hand, when we eat, the stomach becomes full of food. After a full meal, our stomachs become stretched. This is translated into "no need for food now" and the ghrelin cells stops secreting the hormone.

When ghrelin hormone is raised in the blood, it goes to a region in the brain called hypothalamus. A satiety center is located in the hypothalamus. The hormone affects the satiety center so that we feel hungry. Moreover, the stomach and intestine (digestive system – gastrointestinal tract) are getting prepared to receive food. The stomach secretes the acid and the intestine moves in a rhythmic fashion.

In addition, ghrelin inhibits insulin secretion derived by glucose rise. Therefore, the pancreatic cells do not release insulin in the blood allowing glucose to rise. This action is mediated by another hormone called somatostatin. Somatostatin is present in delta cells in the pancreas. The somatostatin cells have receptors that are sensitive to ghrelin. So, when ghrelin docs on these receptors the somatostatin hormone is released and counteract the action of insulin leading to the rise of blood glucose level after meals [130].

It has been postulated that the ghrelin hormone possesses functions other that satiety control. It affects the reward system in the brain including sexual satisfaction. It plays an interesting role in cognitive adaptation to environmental changes [131]. It has an important role in the learning process by acting on memory regions in the brain [132]. Moreover, ghrelin is a strong stimulator of growth hormone [133].

Children with anorexia nervosa (a neurotic disease- the patient doesn't feel hungry and abstain from food to a dangerous level) show high levels of ghrelin hormones in their bodies [134]. Obese children have a low level of ghrelin hormone [135].

The conventional low carb diet makes dieters suffer periods of hunger that keep them lurching from one diet to another. This may end up with a tragic failure to burn fat. This hunger you feel is the result of the increase of blood sugar when you eat and a decrease in blood sugar a few hours later. The ghrelin hormone goes up and down with your meals and hunger pain goes up and down too. Most of the dieters are not happy with that.

On the contrary, when you start a ketogenic diet with high-fat contents and low carbs ghrelin hormone is blocked. This means it will not increase and decrease with your meals. Your body burns fat and you start to notice that you are losing weight.

Ghrelin suppresses the rise of ghrelin that occurs with weight loss. Research studies show that when one eats a high level of ketones more than 0.3mM during dieting, the ghrelin decrease below the baseline level (the level of the hormone before starting a diet) [136]. The decrease of ghrelin hormone helps the dieter to eat less and feel less pain.

More is still, another study shows that the hunger hormone, ghrelin, the level is kept unchanged when the dieter ketone blood level reaches 0.48mM This welcomed effect lasts for 8 weeks of dieting with remarkable weight loss as indicated by the loss of body fat mass [136].

It has been postulated that a blood ketone level of 0.5mM is enough to suppress the ghrelin hormone and stop you feeling hungry [137]. There are several diet regimens that fulfill this target level. We shall discuss the different recipes and alternative meal content choices in detail in the following chapters.

Ketogenic diet and cholesterol

Atherosclerosis (hard & thick artery) is a disease that causes many serious problems such as heart attack due to the coronary artery (arteries of the heart), cerebral stroke, kidney disease, and hypertension. Hardening of the arteries makes the artery to narrow. When the artery becomes narrow, the blood cannot pass easily to its destination. Consequently, the pressure in the artery tends to increase to overcome the narrow segment (s) along the artery course. The resulting increase in pressure is detected by the physician using the sphygmomanometer. The high blood pressure puts you at high risk of various catastrophic events.

Therefore, it is important to take care that your blood has no high level of cholesterol. Low cholesterol level protects you from the deleterious outcome of atherosclerosis. Cholesterol circulates in the blood in various forms such as triglycerides (TG), low-density lipoprotein (LDL), and very low-density lipoprotein (VLDL). You have another cholesterol-carrying protein called high-density lipoprotein (HDL). We also call it the good cholesterol. It is good because it carries the least amount of cholesterol of the other lipoproteins. When the good cholesterol (HDL) is high you are safe. Otherwise, when the bad cholesterol increases (LDL &TG), you should consider some approaches to force them to a lower level.

How does cholesterol harden the arteries and make them narrow? Atherosclerosis initiated when monocytes invade the wall of the artery and turn into macrophages. The macrophage is the eating cell of our defense system. Macrophages derived from monocytes engulf LDL-cholesterol and change to large "foam cells." The foam cells contain many cytoplasmic vesicles and are laden with a high level of fat (lipid).

Then, calcification takes place among vascular smooth muscle cells that are placed in the muscle layer of the arterial wall. Eventually, the cells die with increasing calcium deposition. In addition, the smooth muscle ingests lipids and is replaced by collagen changing into foam cells themselves. A fibrous cap is formed separating the fatty deposits and the artery lining. The fatty deposits and the covering cap are now called *atheroma.*

Accumulating evidence suggests that a ketogenic diet with high fat and low carbs encourages fat burn in the body. The burning of body fat decreases the circulating cholesterol and prevent atheroma formation. LDL-cholesterol is decreased and becomes less likely to be deposited in the arterial wall. Consequently, atheroma is not formed, and the artery remains healthy.

A recent study compared the effect of low-fat diet and low carbs diet on weight loss and serum lipid profile among a group of overweight adolescents. The study concluded that a low-carb diet is very effective in reducing weight on overweight adolescents with safety lipid profile in a short-term study. The low-carbs effect was significantly higher than that of the low-fat diet [138].

Another study proved that low-carbs, high-protein, and high-fat (Atkins) diet results in a remarkable weight loss (4%) more than the conventional diet regimen. The positive effect was noticed in the first 6 weeks. One year follow up showed attrition of adherence in all test groups. This mandate a long-term study to elucidate the long-term safety and efficacy of the Atkins diet [139].

The most recent study supported previous results. The study confirmed that low-carbs weight-loss diet with a high percentage of dietary saturated fat and low refined carbs improves the overall lipid profile of the test group [140].

The accumulating evidence suggests the promising role of ketogenic diet in the management of hypertension, heart stroke, and cerebral stroke that are the direct result of atheroma formation and narrowing of the arterial lumen (arterial stenosis) [141].

Ketogenic diet and athletic performance

For athletes, ketone esters in a syrup form showed improved performance in athletes. Ketosis, activated by high ketone esters, decreases the dependence of the muscles on glycogen storage for production of energy and performance. Instead, muscle cells resort to utilizing ketones and as an alternative source for energy [142].

Even though muscle glycogen is available and insulin in high, the muscle cell utilizes triacylglycerol as an oxidative substrate for energy production. This alternative oxidative pathway sometimes called "the second wind" during which the muscle performs independently of oxygen provided to the cell. The muscle performance increases to a second level when it enters the "second wind" and ketones metabolism is established.

Chapter 8:
Water Fast

What is Water Fast

Water fast is a type of abstinence from food except for water. It is also called water-only fast referring to abstinence from food, tea, juice, noncaloric beverages and any other type of food. Smoking is included in some regimens. The duration of fasting is one to three days only. Fasting regimen of 14 days, for example, mandate medical supervision. Long-time fasting is better practiced under medical supervision not to harm yourself. Several medical empirical studies evaluate the long-term waster-only fasting on the medical problem understudy.

The water-only fast is of benefit in reducing blood pressure to safe levels to maximally reduce the risk of cerebral strokes, coronary heart disease, and hypertension-related kidney disease [143]. Also, water-only fast is proved useful in reducing body weight through restriction of caloric intake [144], [145]. The most characteristic feature of water-only fast is pain reduction in rheumatic disease, thus reducing the doses of corticosteroids and pain killers that have a bad side-effect on the afflicted persons [146].

The research on water-only fast is limited. However, the results that have been obtained so far are promising. It is worth noting that water-only fast would carry some untoward effects on your health. In this section, we try to confer the cones and pros of water-only fast to your hand. This would benefit you to decide what is best for your health and practice it in the right way without hurting yourself.

When we need water-only fast

Health benefit including weight reduction is not the only reason for water-only fast. This type of fast has been practiced since several decades ago for religious and spiritual reasons. However, since proved that the old tradition would confer a great benefit to our health and prevent disease. The ancient wisdom has come to the domain of science to be proved empirically. Also, water fasting is resorted to as a preparatory step before some medical procedures.

Religious water-only fast

Water-fast has been practiced by the Jain principle in India. It is a part of Hinduism and Buddhism. In Jainism, water-fast practice last for 8 to 10 days of the Hindu calendar. Jains believe that fasting increases their spirituality.

Roman Catholicism also observed fasting for spiritual reasons. It is called a eucharistic fast that should be practiced before receiving Eucharist during the Mass. The one who observes fasting, for this reason, should abstain from nutritional and caloric sustenance completely. However, one can still have medicine and drink water. This tradition has become less stringent recently. Another form of fasting that includes water is what is called Black Fast. In Black Fast water and bread are only consumed by monks. Religious individuals who observe Black Fasting believe in practicing mortifications and asceticism. All Catholics, however, are welcome to practice this type of fasting with permission and advice of the spiritual director.

Preparing for medical procedures

any medical procedure that would involve anesthesia (sedation). Some non-sedating procedures may need water fast as preparatory step such as abdominal ultrasound imaging (examining your abdomen using the ultrasound machine). Also, upper gastrointestinal endoscopy needs the person to be totally fast for 8 hours before the procedure.

Health benefits

We can resort to water-only fast for losing weight, detoxing, and as a modality of treatment of certain diseases and pain. We recall that water-only fast with no caloric intake would lead to blood pressure reduction, reducing the pain of rheumatic disease, and enhance autophagy as well.

Juice fast

It is also called a fad diet. In juice, fast water is only consumed, however, in the form of fruit and vegetable juices. This help give taste to water without adding many calories to the diet. One who observer juice fast would abstain from consuming solid food. This type of fasting is used for detoxification. It is also used as alternative medicine. It can be included as a part of detox diets. The diet lasts for two to seven days. It was anecdotally used for promoting health, teat disease, and enhance longevity.

This type of dieting has been challenged by Catherine Collins.[1] Collins stated that detox dieting including juice fast is a marketing myth. There has

---

[1] a chief dietitian of St George's Hospital Medical School, London, England.

been no physiological background for such dieting. She stressed that taking a lot of vitamins, minerals, and laxatives for up to a week has not been proved in any empirical study to be of any health benefit. It is just a marketing myth [147]. On the other hand, Sir Colin Berry, a pathologist advises to let go with detox. Sir Berry said that the great systems of our body have been evolved over thousands of year. Our body knows well how to get rid of the harming stuff and detox would help. He also advised drinking fewer beverages.

Water fast for hypertension

Goldhamer and colleagues conducted a study to empirically evaluate the effect of a water-only fast on the level of hypertension [143]. Dr. Goldhamer has proposed a scientific regimen for water-only fast for a long period of 40 days. The volunteered were under strict medical supervision.

They found that the blood pressure was reduced significantly to the level of 110/70 mmHg. At this blood pressure level, we have the minimum risk to develop cerebral stroke, heart attacks, and kidney disease.

Water-fast for weight reduction

A research study conducted in China proved that 7-days fasting has a potential role in preventing metabolic syndrome including obesity [148]. This study, also, suggests the deployment of this regiment as a treatment option in metabolic syndromes. However, further studies are needed before finally establishing 7-day fasting as a therapeutic regimen.

The study showed that fasting was the cause of 5.5% weight reduction with the enhanced effect of glucose regulation, cardiac metabolites, and the endocrine profile. The affected endocrine profile includes leptin-to-adiponectin ratio that is related to insulin sensitivity.

It is worth noting that the 7-days fasting was not associated with relevant hunger or side effects. Moreover, it has been observed that water-only fast exerts a positive impaction of mood with antidepressant and anxiety relieving impactions. The blood pressure and lipid profile were also improved.

Water-only fast regimens from research

The following regimens are used by the physician in their research work and proved effective and safe. They can be adopted by you. Medical supervision is needed for long term fasting, more than 3 days. The researchers used these regiment for longer periods of fasting. The lengthy fasting is not recommended without medical consultation and supervision.

Before being set on the water-only fast regimen, one should start with a preparatory diet. The preparatory diet consists of fresh raw fruits and vegetables and steamed vegetables. This step is an important transition before starting the proper fast. With the sole exception of pure water, you should abstain from all food and beverages. You may restrict your activities to reading, writing, taking educational courses, or online activities. Strenuous exercise is not recommended. You can listen to music instead.

You can continue as such for up to 3 days with no harm. After 3 days, there will be a period of refeeding. During refeeding, you would have juices made from fresh raw fruits and vegetables. You are allowed to receive up to 12 ounces of fresh juice every 3 hours. The juice phase would last for one day to be followed by eating sold fruits and vegetables. Finally, the whole natural food is reintroduced [143].

Another clinically proved regiment by Chinese researcher lasts for 7 days. The preparatory (transition) days constitutes of 2 days on 800Kcal only with low-calories and low-salt intake. You can obtain these calories from pure cooked rice and vegetables-Chinese food. During the fasting period, you should abstain from all foodstuffs. You are allowed to have herbal tea without any limitations. Also, you can have 200 calories of fruit juice and small standard quantities of light vegetable soup. The max daily caloric intake should not exceed 300 Kcal.

The emptiness of the bowel was achieved by the end of the preparatory days. A 30-40 g sodium sulfate, as a laxative, was used for bowel emptying. This step is important to slow down the intestinal motility to avoid retarded and unfavorable digestion. Therefore, the initiation of water-only fast would not be associated with bowel symptoms.

The Chinese model of water-only fast allows for 2-3 liter of fluid each day.

Finally, at the end of the 7-days fasting period, you can revert to the low-calorie diet for 3 consecutive days. The solid food should be back to your diet gradually. Caffeine and alcoholic beverages should not be consumed during the fasting regimen.

Buchinger fasting regimen

Buchinger (1878-1966) was the first scientist who designed a therapeutic fasting regimen for weight reduction based on scientific evidence. It was first called therapeutic fasting (also Heilfast). The medically supervised, inpatient multidisciplinary fasting regimen proposed by Buchinger can be used for disease prevention as well as therapeutic purposes.

The traditional Buchinger fasting is founded on a daily intake of vegetables. One should receive the only 0.25L of vegetable broth and the same amount of fruits or vegetable juice. Honey is allowed in 30g. Fluid intake was nearly 2.5L in the form of herbal teas and water. Buttermilk was added to the regimen by Fahrner in fasting for longer periods [149].

The fasting was practicing in groups of people sharing the same experience together. Fasting in groups is of psychosocial benefits rather than observing fasting alone. The evolved spiritual dimension is shown to be characterized by enhancement of spiritual practice with improved access to a higher level of consciousness. The positive mental effect is presumed to be the target of all world religions.

Buchinger proposed fasting to have medial physiological therapeutic dimension as well. The three domains/dimensions act synergistically and should not be split apart. During the fasting period, one is encouraged to practice music, painting, meditation, or reading. It is called the dietetics of the soul by Buchinger.

Intermittent Fasting

The principle of intermittent fasting has been established by two physicians, Edward Hooker Dewey, American physician, (1837–1904) and Guillaume Guelpa, a French physician, (1850–1930). Dr. Dewey favored daily fasting. The duration of fasting ends at late noon. His pioneer work starts in the USA in the late 19th century. Thanks to his sincere work, the notion of health advantages from cyclic caloric restriction has been propagated and further intensified by science. Dr. Guelpa is a French physician in the early 20th century, who designed continuing cycles of fasting for 2-5 days. After the fasting period, one should continue on vegetarian food for12-15 days.

Extensive experimental research on calorie restriction leads to the establishment of the principle of intermittent fasting (also called alternative fasting). Moreover, intermittent fasting has been introduced into human clinical research and medical practice. It has been approved by the scientific community.

The well-established regimens include alternate fasting day (AFD) where diet is served every other day (every-other-day diet) [150]. Another regimen depends on scheduled fasting and eating days with 5 days eating and 2 days fasting or 25 days eating and 5 days fasting [151]. These regimens are used currently with great success in achieving the goals.

During the eating time/days, you can consume food as well as water (ad libitum). In the fasting days, food is either restricted or withheld completely; you maintain on water only.

The initial studies postulated that intermittent fasting can reduce the risk of type 2 diabetes and heart disease. The fasting regimen was suggested to play a role in the management of cancer. However, further research is needed to elucidate these promising domains.

Other water-only fast regimens

F.X. Mayer therapy

F.X. Mayer, an Austrian physician, has developed a water-only fasting approach in 3 steps. The first step is tea and water-only fasting. The second step is low-calorie milk-bread diet. The third one is a mild intestinal diet that is poor in fibers.

Johann Schroth approach

Johann Schroth (1798-1856), an Austrian naturopath, has designed a calorie-restricted vegetarian diet. The proposed diet by Schroth was rich in carbs. Water-fast days was alternating with days of restricted fluid intake. Schroth allowed 500ml of white wine.

Whet cure

This procedure is supplemented with whey. Whey is a protein-rich milk product. As an alternative, oatmeal or buckwheat gruel can be given to subjects as a supplement. The nutrition energy intake was 500 Kcal/d.

Chapter 9:
Myths and autophagy

How do we get information about dieting?

We usually get our information about dieting from fitness magazines, mainstream books, and forums. We may also follow a friend's advice or speculations on the medial. The social networks are also a source for out information. No one would bother going to a dietitian specialist or a physician before making a diet decision.

Likewise, a bunch of dietary myths runs rampant in the fitness and dieting community. These myths are just believed because we hear them form celebrities or bodybuilders. We never give us a break and ask a specialist or search deep to find the truth. We are now busy and tired!

Close scrutiny reveals that most of the widespread myths are built on half-truths or faulty conclusions. Some myths are built on false science that is rejected by the true scientific community. Commercials push sales for certain supplements or nutrients because one or two preliminary studies have said so and so. Other myths are a mere creation of our mind that tries to overcome gaps of information,

In the following section, we will stress on the myths related to autophagy and the scientific bases behind each notion. When scientific research is lacking, we will say so.

Stick to the basic

- Autophagy, as the name implies, is a degradation process. The body destroys the old items to build a new one.

- Autophagy is triggered by energy deprivation. Energy deprivation means abstinence from eating a high caloric diet including carbs and fats.

- Deprivation of energy activates a cell sensor, thus allowing autophagy to run.

- Fasting, which means low glucose (calorie) intake, causes insulin level in our blood to decrease to the basal level, at which autophagy is initiated. Therefore, eating much sugar or sugary diet will cause insulin to rising and autophagy to seize.

- Moreover, protein-rich diet will release amino acids into the blood. The synthesis of glucose from protein sources is activated and autophagy stops.

- Only caloric restriction and fasting are the only known proved way to promote autophagy.

What is true and what is false?

1. Fruit and coffee and autophagy

It has been claimed that fruit does not break autophagy. Fruit supplies us with fructose. It is a sugar similar to glucose. Like glucose, fructose can be metabolized by the liver and stored as glycogen. When the glycogen stores in the liver are replenished, metabolism reverts away from using fat and ketone bodies. Bodies shifts back to use glycogen as a source for energy instead.

Fruits are good for health. Fruits would keep your catabolic state but not autophagy. That is to say that autophagy would not keep you in a fasted state of autophagy for sure.

You have to realize the fact that you can be in a solid state of autophagy and keep your muscle bulk. The reverse is true.

Now, what about coffee. Coffee does not break your fast of autophagy. On the contrary, coffee can promote autophagy and enhance ketosis. Coffee seeds contain polyphenols [152] that would stimulate autophagy. In the animal model, autophagy was observed one to 4 hours after coffee consumption. Autophagic flux was observed in all organs subjected to the study namely the liver, muscle, and heart [153]. Caffeine promotes lipolysis of fatty acids with the lowering of insulin and enforcing ketosis.

However, you have to drink coffee devoid of any sugary additives such as milk, cream, or sweeteners. These additives counteract coffee effect by increasing insulin level and halts fast for autophagy.

2. You need 3-5 days fast to start autophagy.

You need to induce energy deprivation and fasting in one way and not the only way to trigger autophagy. The statement has some truth. One has to fast for at least 3 hours to trigger autophagy and enter into ketosis state. The dropped fact is that autophagy is a balance between two sensors in the cells (mTOR and AMPK).

When you maintain on a diet that is low in carb, moderate in protein, and high in fat content, you will receive small energy reserves and you are ready to enter the therapeutic zone as early as possible. In spite you still actually eating food, your body has no energy supplies. The body will turn to consume the stored energy supplies. That is to say, the body is going to "eat itself." Now, autophagy begins.

3. Autophagy is activated within 24 hours

The calculation of one hour is misleading. The 24 hours relies on research work and animal models and not on the true human circumstances. It is a half-true statement. When you start fasting, your body does not. Actually, your body is busy digesting, absorbing, and metabolizing the last meals. Severn to eight hours should pass before the body starts to "feel" in need of energy.

After the elapse of 20 hours, your body has been in the fasting state for 12 hours only. This time period is not enough for autophagy to be triggered. Actually, a minimum of 3 days and a maximum of 5 days are needed for autophagy to be triggered provided that you are maintained on low carb, high-fat diet.

However, the fasting period is not without benefit. Your insulin level will go down. The inflammation is reduced. Other hormonal levels are readjusted.

4. Activate Autophagy very often

When you fast for three days or maintain on a low-carb, low-fat diet, your body will get benefit from autophagy. Like this, autophagy will fight cancer cells. The cells with old DNA, abnormal protein aggregates, and infected by certain viruses will be destroyed by autophagy. Immunity will be boosted with autophagy as well to combat infections. The old skin cells , fibroblast, will be destroyed to be replaced by new cells. Therefore, the aging facial feature will be delayed. And so on.

On the other hand, autophagy can do exactly the opposite. For example, Brucella species are replicated and grow using cell autophagy. Hepatitis C virus is replicated and multiplicated using the autophagy proteins as triggers to turn the process to the visionbenefit. Although Beclin 1 protein has been proved to be involved in tumor suppression, Beclin 1 protein can help some types of cancer to survive. Last but not least, repeated autophagy would direct the body to utilize muscle proteins as a source of energy. The net result is muscle wasting and weakness.

The good practice is that you practice autophagy fasting less often to get the best out of the procedure. Prolonged or extensive autophagy stimulation may lead to the emergence of untoward or unexpected (under investigation) side effects. Intermittent fasting or autophagy is considered the best practice to get the benefits and avoid harm. Autophagy is a way to get healthy, not diseased. It is not a diet cult either. You have a long life to enjoy.

5. Exercise compromises autophagy

On the contrary, exercise induces autophagy. Exercise makes your cells more sensitive to autophagy. When you exercise, the effect of the ketone diet is exaggerated.

Experimental study on animal models revealed that exercise could decrease the level of beta-amyloid in the brain cells. Accumulation of beta-amyloid is responsible for Alzheimer's disease in humans. The exercise was found to activate autophagy and hence, the reduction of the level of amyloid deposition [154].

Moreover, exercise is responsible for modifying muscle cell metabolism (myofibrils) and enhancing the contractile properties of the skeletal muscles. One empirical study proved that exercise send signals to autophagy to start. Activation of autophagy has been proved to perform metabolic adaptation to exercise [155].

Therefore, it has been suggested that autophagy fast can be combined with exercise for maximum autophagy activation and consequently, muscle growth. So, the speculation that exercise stops autophagy is completely untrue.

6. Autophagy equals starvation

It is not a precise statement. Autophagy is not starvation is not precise either. In fact, starvation is when your body is derived of the external as well as internal energy stores like in famines. Autophagy is an internal procedure by which the body consumes fast, stored in our body, instead of glucose and other sugars. Fat consumption will create ketone state that is good for reducing weight and combat atherosclerosis and other degenerative diseases.

Moreover, autophagy consumes the old cells, organelles, and proteins for producing energy. This process is a useful recycling process. Cell recycling helps destroy the bad cells and hopes for the creation of new ones. The consequent result is to ride of cancer cells and renewal of skin cells. This effect has a direct impact on longevity and health.

When you perceive autophagy as a way of renewing and refreshing your body, you are looking to the positive side. Starvation is a wrong way to approach it, especially as it is a process that should not be done very often. Thoughts are very important to direct our behavior and emotions. We should focus mindset and emotions on the positive.

<u>7. **Muscles are built by autophagy.**</u>

Building new muscle cells is an energy consuming process. You need the energy to synthesize proteins and then, use this protein to synthesize new muscle cells or muscle fibers. Autophagy, on the contrary, is a catabolic (degenerating) process. Hardly, one can combine the degenerating and regenerating process under the same dietary condition.

The solid fact is that autophagy consumes protein aggregates in the cell, old organelles, and broken structures. The resulting amino acids are used to synthesize new proteins and organelles for the cells. However, we should not jump to the conclusion that autophagy enhances muscle building.

Generating a new muscle is a different story. You need to provide your body with the essential amino acids (these are amino acids that are not generated by the body and must be given by food) like leucine to build the muscle proteins. These amino acids are derived from food. When you are on diet or fasting, how would you get the essential amino acids on regular bases for building muscles?

8. Autography helps to remove loose skin

"autophagy can eat up loose skin" is really a myth and a marketing tactic. "Autophagy tightens up loose skin after losing a bunch of weight" is a deceiving phrase.

The only fact that comes from true research work tells us that fibroblast cells are responsible for collagen disposition in our skin. Old fibroblasts generate collagen in the skin. Accumulation of collagen causes the aging appearance of skin wrinkling and looseness. Autophagy keeps fibroblasts health and removes the old ones. Therefore, collagen will not accumulate in the skin. No one talks about loose skin or redundancy. This fact has been used to trick people to believe some commercials.

The truth is fasting and hence, autophagy may reduce the progression of loosening of the skin when weight is successfully reduced. When one loses much weight, wrinkling and looseness of the skin are inevitable. However, autophagy can minimize this process. autophagy keeps the skin healthy and young rather than tightening it. Therefore, calorie restriction without autophagy would cause more loose skin than when autophagy is activated.

It should be acknowledged that the skin condition is kept from collagen disposition as long as possible. This will give us a younger look. However, the media and marketing would exaggerate the truth to push sales.

9. Autophagy is not halted by fat

Insulin is released from the beta cells of Langerhans' islets when the blood sugar, namely glucose, or amino acids level raises in blood. High level of fat or cholesterol in the blood would not stimulate insulin release. Therefore, eating a high-fat diet would not stimulate insulin secretion. However, you can still go to a fed state by consuming fat.

The fat diet promotes ketosis. Ketosis promotes macroautophagy in the brain by activating Sirt 1 and hypoxia-inducible factor 1 [110]. In addition, ketone bodies elicit chaperone-mediated autophagy that targets specific amino acids and substrates [156]. Ketones are increased in the blood during fasting and when you eat a ketonic diet as well.

The mTOR (mammalian target of rapamycin) responds to any calorie excess, not only glucose and amino acids. Therefore, ketones can inhibit autophagy through mTOR. So, fat-rich diet slows down autophagy and does not cause complete cessation. However, excessive fat intake (more than

100 calories) would enforce autophagy to stop. Diet will not get so high to stop autophagy. We recall that you should be well informed about autophagy because too much and too less is harmful or not beneficial.

10. Branched-chain amino acids do not stop autophagy

When you reach this level in the book, you will find this statement a complete myth. Branched-chain amino acids contain pure amino acids. Amino acids will absolutely block autophagy. Only small amounts are needed to achieve this effect.

Elevation of ketosis saves muscles from eating themselves. Ketosis provides an energy source other than protein and amino acids. This will keep the muscle intact. If your diet is poor in protein and another nutrient, you are at risk of stopping autophagy and losing muscle mass. The branched-chain amino acids will shift the body into a fed state and inhibit ketosis. Thus, autophagy is stopped and you will get no benefit out of this. The branched-chain amino acids are not needed in your diet.

11. Eating meat is against autophagy

This myth sounds like if you eat meat you will be deprived of autophagy for your lifetime and you will be cursed with aging. The most important thing in autophagy is the frequency of your meals. Even with protein restriction, you will not get autophagy as long as you don't last long enough – 3 days at least.

For your understanding, practicing intermittent fasting will drive autophagy to work irrespective to your protein diet at the eating period. Similarly, when you are a fully plant-based vegan diet and you eat frequently, you will not have autophagy stimulated.

So, it is the fasting days, not exactly the content of the food that would stimulate autophagy. That is why intermittent fasting propagates from the nineteenth century till now.

Water fasting and Autophagy

Water fasting is a type of fasting that restricts an individual to drinking and living on water for a number of hours. This method has become very popular in recent years as it has proven to be a shortcut to making individual lose weight. However water fasting is only practiced between 24-72 hours except under strict medical supervision. When water fasting is prolonged, it loses complications on the health of animals. It may lead to exacerbation of malnourishment and dysfunction, especially in old and aging subjects.

There have been established facts that support the notion that water fasting promotes and helps to promote autophagy. Although, these research methods have not fully scored on human, except on mice. A group of scientists carried out a profound experiment on the effect of fasting on autophagy [180]. They opined that the subjection of animals to water fasting led to a dramatic neuronal autophagy regulation. This change was prompted by the abrupt increase in auto phagosome and lowered activity of neuronal mTOR.

Water fasting has shown a great deal of commitment in ensuring metabolism and change in cellular activities that may affect inflammation and metabolism energy optimization [181,182,183,184].

Ketosis and Autophagy

Having laid notable facts about ketosis and Autophagy and treated them explicitly in previous chapters, the two bio-independent processes however have strong connective links. However, these processes only support each other and are not inclusive, mutually. Ketosis can be achieved without phasing through autophagy and also can autophagy be achieved without a need to undergo ketosis. They can only be seen together in most cases as a result of similar principles they both exhibit.

Do you need Ketosis to activate Autophagy?

The bio-scientific processes of Autophagy and Ketosis are regulated by a couple of factors:

- Deprivation of energy due to fasting, physical exercise, thermoregulation, insufficient supply of amino acid and glucose. In metabolic processes, low amount of insulin is needed to be produced, so also mTOR. However, AMPK is required in high proportion.

- Subjection of the human body to glucose restriction fastens the process of ketosis and makes the process easily achieved. There are two primary bio-processes that usually lead to the production of keto bodies in the human body. The first is when carbohydrate is consumed deficiently. Ketones require low-carbs diets before they are produced in the body. On the other hand, depletion of liver glycogen could also lead to ketone bodies production.. Also, through a process called Glucogenesis, protein can be synthesized. Although, this process is a secondary process and does not really affect ketosis in such noticeable way. For this, mTOR and insulin may not be required, even though it is unlikely to occur.

The human body can achieve ketosis by consuming high level of mTOR and high proportion of insulin because of high concentration of protein and amount of calories consumed. This will lead to eventual elevation of ketone bodies and maintenance of nutritional ketosis. Although, this will halt Autophagy as a result of high concentration of nutrients embed in mTOR.

Contrary to many people's belief, Autophagy does not need ketosis to become activated. You can fast for three days and yet not be in ketosis (depending on how committed you are to keto diet). But to achieve ketosis, certain Autophagy prerequisites must have been met. Such prerequisites include low blood glucose, mTOR and insulin.

Autophagy and ketone measurement

It takes an average of 48-72 hours fasting before autophagy gets activated. However, the length of time is determined by the nutrient composition of an individual based on mTOR AMPK kinase. The nutrient status of the body of an individual accounts for how long autophagy will take to activate in the body. The presence of amino acids, ketones and glucose plays vital role in activating autophagy.

In general, there are no standard methods of measuring autophagy in the human body but can be estimated by the insulin-glucagon ratio and glucose ketone index.

> - If insulin level is higher compared to glucagon level, it suggests more anabolism, higher insulin, nutrient presence and hugged blood sugar.
> - If insulin level is lower compared to glucagon level, it indicates more catabolism, gluconeogenesis, nutrient deprivation and fat oxidation.
> - The index of glucagon ketone is used to estimate the insulin-glucagon ratio.

However, if the index gives a low computational output, higher ketosis and more AMPK are implied.

How to calculate Glucose-Ketone index (GKI)

1. Take a measurement of your blood glucose.
2. Take also the measurement of the amount of ketones in your body.
3. Divide the output in (I) by 18
4. Divide the result in (III) by the figure measured in (II)

However, if mg/dl is used as the unit of glucose level, the third step may be discarded.

Prevention of age-related complications and lifespan expansion via starvation

In 1917, a researcher reported that restriction on calorie intake can spontaneously help to increase life longevity and slow down growth rate [185]. However, the result of the research was put forward but was unfortunately rejected by many people because the researcher failed to provide detailed explanation on the methodological processes adopted while carrying out his research. Fast forward to 1935, another scientist, MacCay, came on board to publish a research paper showing caloric restriction in rats can help to increase lifespan. The same pattern of research was carried out successfully on human beings.

During the Second World War, there was obvious deprivation of calorie intake, and this restriction has contributed to the human health effectively. In Europe, the World War II led to people having just little food to consume and it resulted in anti-aging benefits. As a result of this, there were reduced cases of hypertension, heart complications and diabetes recorded. In addition, only a few records were made about cancer. Amongst the Norwegian women, the incidence of cancer recorded was far lower than the general expectation during the season of food shortage (World War II).

Roles of Keto diets and Autophagy in ensuring lifespan extension

Keto diets can make a dieter live up to a century, not because keto diets are clinically proven to improve overall health but because the process is phased through a physiological process known as Autophagy. In autophagy, normal physiological processes occur where the cells in the human body devour themselves. This may sound scary but it is completely an healthy and normal process. During the process of autophagy, the cells in the human body are made to dissemble damaged and unnecessary parts of the body and recycle the parts that are still much functioning. Autophagy generally improves health, make cells function better and the effect of this is increased longevity.

In several past studies, it has been established that ketone bodies are useful in up regulating autophagy [186]. Meanwhile, eating diets with more carbohydrate proportion and being physically inactive tend to down-regulate the process of autophagy which subsequently accelerates aging process. This happens as a result of the tendency of the human cells to accumulate all damaged body organelles and proteins during metabolism. Autophagy make properly-functioning and healthy cells only when metabolism is not in action.

Summarily, autophagy is only achieved with the aid of healthy diets and dedicated lifestyle. Up regulating autophagy process through ketogenic dietary helps to improve the overall health which subsequently helps with this cycling program.

Ketone and anti-aging process

The most crucial aspect of aging is the vascular aging. As human beings get older, the vessels that supply the body parts with essential nutrients become more sensitive, weaker and more susceptible to aging damage. Hence, the need to place more emphasis on vascular aging. In the human body, a compound called Beta-hydroxybutyrate is produced. This compound is a ketone and is produced in the liver as molecule during the period of starvation, fasting and when an individual is on low-carb diets. Beta-hydroxybutyrate compound promotes multiplication and division of cells that line the interior surface of blood vessels. Cell division is however a clear indication of anti-aging process, simultaneously serving as marker for cellular youth. This ketone produced by the liver delays the aging of endothelial cells, which are found in blood vessels. The compound is found to prevent senescence, a type of cellular aging.

Keto diets and weight loss

Weight loss

When the body system is subjected to carbohydrate deficiency or total deprivation for a few days, ketones are produced in the body. Ketones are alternative sources that provide the brain and nervous systems with fuel while they simultaneously aid weight loss. When the body enters ketosis and starts burning ketones for fuel, the dieter will experience and increase in energy level and decreased appetite. This results in consumption of fewer calories and subsequent weight loss.

The link between ketone and ketosis is not far-fetched. Ketones are known to have mild diuretic effects on dieters. Most of the times, people mistaken this process of weight loss for a completely different reason. Weight loss is sometimes interpreted as if it results from fat. In actual fact, the rapid weight loss in the first seven days of keto diet is as a result of water loss from the body.

<u>Rapid weight loss</u>

Keto diet is one of the most effective ways of losing weight rapidly and burn fat. In the first week of ketogenic dieting, the dieter experiences a rapid weight loss from around 2 to 10 pounds. This figure can only be achieved by subjecting oneself to keto diets. There are scientific researches that have proven it that no other diet can give such drastic change. In actual fact, this drastic weight loss occurs as a result of the body shedding the extra water weight it held on to from carbohydrate consumption. Occasionally, the experience is followed by flu-like symptoms. This is why it is important to always drink a lot of water when you're on ketogenic diets.

After the first week, the rate of weight loss slows down and is steadily maintained throughout the period of keto dieting. During this period, the body tries to adapt to the new diet change and subsequently switches from burning of carbohydrates to burning of fats.

<u>How fast does weight loss occur with keto diets?</u>

Once you leap the first week of ketogenic dieting and successfully proceeds to ketosis, fat starts to burn off your system (provided you have calorie deficit). At this stage, the rate of weight loss is reduced to an average of 1-2 pounds weekly.

As you approach your weight goal and your body weight reduces, the rate of weight loss is slowed down. This occurs because weight loss demands more calories. As a result of this, there's probably a need for you to check your calorie level, at the end of every month.

It is worth noting that keto diet weight loss is not always consistent. It may appear like you haven't lost a pound weight in a week, and when you eventually check, you realize that you have lost about 3-4 pounds.

Factors that determine the rate of weight loss

Health status:

The current health status of a dieter plays a leading role in determining how fast or how slow weight loss would occur and how such dieter should adapt to the new (low-carb diet) system. If a dieter has any hormone-related or metabolic problems, weight loss might occur at a very slow rate and more challenging than expected. For example, excess visceral fat, thyroid problems and insulin resistance can leave a tremendous impact on the rate at which the body loses weight.

Calorie deficit:

This is the most significant factor responsible for the rate of weight loss. Simply put, it determines how consistent the process occurs. When only few calories are consumed than the minimum amount required by the body system, weight loss occurs. This implies that your weight loss increases as calorie consumption decreases. Although, there's always a need to regulate calorie deficit. The human body has a natural way of preventing massive weight loss during starvation via mechanisms that allow long-term fat loss much harder to achieve and maintain. This is why it is not a good idea to subject the body to prolonged starvation. Researches show that calorie deficit above the line 30% is well enough to stimulate some of these mechanisms for long-term fat loss.

Daily habits:

The daily habits of a dieter tell if the efforts channeled at weight loss are appreciative or equal total waste. In keto dieting, a dieter is expected to remain consistent to achieve the weight loss goal. Such dieter must learn to eat clean keto foods. There is also a need to avoid high-fat junk foods with low quality ingredients for success to be in view. In addition to all of these, a dieter is primarily required to watch-out for hidden carbs in diets and ensure daily and consistent exercise. These daily habits, together with right amount of foods will help foster the weight loss goal, and makes the dieter achieve a successful body transformation.

Body composition:

Body composition is yet another important factor that plays a vital role in determining how fast pounds come off. If a dieter has more pounds to shred, the process happens faster than in dieters with just a few extra pounds to burn off their bodies. The best analysis of this can be explained by the fact that obese people can maintain a much larger calorie deficit easily, which eventually leads to faster weight loss. The mass of the muscle also plays a role. Muscle mass helps to keep the metabolic rate of a dieter from dropping significantly as weight reduces. The effect of this is revealed in the stabilization of weight loss rate and may also lead to prevention of a dreaded weigh loss plateau.

When the rate of weight loss is properly checked, some patterns begin to emerge. For instance, people who lose weight slowly while on KD are those with poor metabolic health, bad eating habits and lack of adequate exercise. On the other hand, dieters that begin with more muscles and decent metabolic health and are discipline enough to maintain their diet plans maintain calorie deficit, and subsequently increase the level of their physical activities.

Generally, people are naturally integrated with different lifestyle and health, which implies that the rate of weight loss of each individual will be different. In spite of the differences, if the diets are consistently maintained, our body will change to our desired configuration.

How much weight is lost when you follow keto diets?

Keto diets work effectively if they are well-formulated and strictly followed. Every body has a potential to sculpt into incredible shape with keto diets. However, not everyone will achieve the desired body shape goal by simply being in ketosis and on low carbs.

Discussing from a dietary perspective, consistency, discipline, well-formulated and healthy dietary are the needed basics to getting the body shape you desire.

To get started on weight loss journey, there are some basic principles required of every dieter to formulate healthy keto diet:

➢ A keto dieter must ensure that right amount of protein and calories are consumed than meet the weight loss goal.

- A keto dieter must ensure that most of the calories consumed are derived from macronutrient dense foods.
- A keto dieter must ensure that the diet objectively and subjectively improves his/her overall health and well-being.
- A keto dieter must be able to adjust his/her lifestyle to suit the weight loss goal.

How to know you're following a well-formulated and healthy keto diet

There have been a number of researches on the effects of diets on mental health and general well-being of human. However, a few established facts are culled out to be benefits

Energy level improvement:

Feeling motivated and energetic is a common effect of keto diet. It has been reported by many people that ketogenic diets improve alertness as well as making dieters more proactive.

Improved stress response:

On a long-term basis, keto diet makes a dieter feel calmer and less-stressed.

Relevant biomarkers:

The levels of blood pressure, triglyceride, blood sugar and cholesterol improve on a well-formulated keto diet.

Better mood:

Ketogenic dieters are reported to feel happier and more optimistic. This is related to the absence of the negative effect of sugar on mental health.

Confidence boost:

Loosing weight on keto diets and getting healthier gives more confidence boost and make a dieter feel generally better.

Keto diets and abdominal fat

The worst type of fat is the abdominal fat. It is notoriously difficult to get rid of, in the human body. Researches have revealed the strong link between abdominal fats and cardiovascular diseases, diabetes and heart attack [171]. There were also evidential facts tabled to corroborate that belly fats are liable to increase the risk of cancer, brain tumor and allergies [172].

However, keto diets and change of lifestyle can help shoot down the risk of having abdominal fats. Keto diets are known to burn fats instead of storing them, which makes them uniquely right for stubborn abdominal fat. Belly fats, subsequently leading to abdominal obesity, are easy to denote in human, especially when the circumference of the waist is above 35 inches and 30 inches in men and women respectively [173].

Loosing abdominal fats with easy steps

Cut down on carb intake

Cutting down on carb and especially processed sugar will quickly aid belly-fat-burning process. Processed sugar has a high nutritional portion of fructose. Fructose is a type of simple sugar which several studies have proven to aid increase of cardiovascular disease risk, as well as type II diabetes [174]. Compared to other studies, fructose has higher probability of causing formation of fats below the visceral line of the stomach [175] which results in pot-belly. However, sugar is not the only problem that needs be avoided. Complex carbs must be cut down since all carbs can lead to weight gain [176]. Unless carb intake is cut down, there will always be problems when you want to lose belly fats.

The ketosis diet decreases the mass of carb intake below 50g daily. The result of this is that the body switches to ketosis. During this phase, the body is forced to burn fats stored as fuel because carbs cannot be used for that purpose. In order to keep carb consumption low on keto diets, about 65-80% of fat, moderate amount of protein and low-carb is needed as nutritional composition of keto diets required to burn abdominal fats.

Consume more fats

It may sound counter-intuitive to say that eating more fats will help to burn out fats. In 2015, a study was carried out on people who were on low-carb and high-fats diets, and results showed that people on high-fat diets lost more fats than those on low-fat diets [177]. In the conducted research, 4.4% of total mass of body weight was lost after 8 weeks of high-fat diet intake.

Fat is essentially required to keep the body full when you are on ketogenic diet because and also needed for ketone production. However, not all types of fats have equal satiating effect. MCTs are the most satiating type of fats, and that is why it is much required as part of keto diet [178].

Monounsaturated fatty acids derived from Olive oil have unsaturated and satiating fatty acids. There is an evidence that when fiber-rich foods and fats are eaten together, satiety increases. However, satiety is not the sole factor needed for belly fat burn. It only provides the energy needed by the body to burn calories. In fact, fats are proven to contain 9calories per gram, which makes them the most powerful energy source.

Consume enough protein

Ketogenic diets are recommended with moderate intake of protein. Protein takes about 0.8-1.6g per kg of total weight of the body [179]. This implies that if your weight is 70kg, your body can take up to 50g often protein daily.

Protein is an essential body-building and muscle-building food. It is the most satiating of all keto macros. This is why it is commonly said that protein helps to control appetite. During metabolism process of protein, the body burns lots of calories as a result of the energy required to break down protein molecules.

Many body tissues, including the muscle are made up of protein. It is essentially important to build muscles in order to burn abdominal fats. This is because the mass of the muscle increases RMR and expends more energy. Muscles aid the body composition you're yearning for.

However, going crazy on protein would only exacerbate the health situation. Keto diet emphasizes that protein should be consumed moderately. When protein is consumed in excess, the body metabolizes extra protein, processes it into a metabolic process commonly referred to as gluconeogenesis. The effect of this is that the dieter is kicked out of ketosis, which is not palatable for anyone aiming at burning abdominal fats.

Chapter 10:
The go home message

Here we conclude the pearls of the book for easy memorization. We will summarize the solid facts and promises of autophagy for future use and benefits. There is no shade of doubt that the research on autophagy is still immature, albeit progressing. Everyday, a new research result is added to support the benefit of autophagy on evidence-based scientific ground. Stimulation of autophagy doesn't need chemicals or artificial martials. Modifications of the way we eat is enough to keep our bodies on the healthy track.

A. Autophagy is a natural process in your body for regeneration and renewal of the cells and their components. It is a dynamic process that carries great potentials in treating degenerative disease, beating aging, reducing weight.

B. Autophagy was proved to treat many of the degenerative disease of the brain and vessels. However, the experiment is still at animal model levels. We should not jump to the conclusions. Everything will come at ease.

being a natural feeding habit without use of chemical materials increases the safety profile of the regimens.

C. Autophagy diet are suggested to enhance autophagy process. The on-going research support the principles; however, the regimens are anecdotal.

D. Ketone diet depends on providing our bodies with low-carbs, moderate amount of proteins, and high-fat diet. This composition proves effective in enforcing the metabolism of our bodies to utilize ketones as a source of energy instead of glucose. Fat is, then, mobilized from the fat stores leading to weight reduction.

E. You have to practice intermittent fast under the supervision of your dietitian. It is better to know that fasting may not be suitable for a subset of people. An expert opinion should be counselled first.

F. Beware of getting information from people other than expertise and licensed personnel. You need someone to coach you first before going on by yourself.

Autophagy carries a promising hope for patients with Alzheimer's disease, Parkinson's disease, atherosclerosis, and more. Now, we have hope that those destructive untreatable disease would be managed by just changing the way we eat.

Fasting was an ancient tradition, however, science proves that not all the traditions are myths. Some of ancient traditions carries great benefit to humans. Many plants that was used by these traditions are proved beneficial to humans by the Western empirical science. However, we have to be a pit caution when we are offered to use herbals or plant extracts. A few of these can be harmful to you while tolerable by others.

Intermittent fasting has been suggested by American and French scientists in the 19th and 20th century respectively. Since then, the accumulating body of evidence proves the efficacy of this regimen in treating many diseases with no harm. However, the duration of the regimen ranged from 3 to 40 days and the diet was carried under the close supervision of expert physicians. The presence of medical supervision is mandatory to ensure safety and prevent harm.

We hope that this book illuminated the path of autophagy to the way of health and fitness. We aimed to provide you with the true scientific information that are deeply rooted in the ground of empirical evidences and away of myths and deception.

Everyday, there is a new light guiding us to the right way. We hope this book would be the new light of today.

30 easy keto diet recipes

Keto diet is such an amazing way to reduce blood pressure, improve your energy level and also maintain constant level of insulin.

1. Paleo keto bread

Keto diet beginners are usually have worries about missing out on delicious diets, and more specifically, the delicious carby goodness of bread. Paleo keto bread is totally different. It has all that you need, delicious and promotes good health.

Ingredients:

- Coconut flour
- Almond flour
- Egg whites
- Baking powder
- Butter

Instructions:

- Mix all dry ingredients together in a food processor, then add some melted butter.
- Beat the egg whites until very stiff peaks, pulse in just half, then fold whatever remains. The aim of beating the egg whites is to allow

the bread have air pockets and some fluffiness.

- Take the mixed ingredients, transfer to (non-sticky) baking pan and bake in an oven regulated between 325-350 degrees Fahrenheit.

There are optional ingredients that could be added in baking Paleo bread. They are cream of tartar, erythritol and xanthan gum. The cream of tartar enables you to achieve stiff peaks easily while you are beating egg whites. The erythritol is there to give the bread some sweetness every white bread does have. Since it is a natural sweetness, it can be included but coconut sugar is a better Paleo ingredient in place of erythritol. Xanthan gum is barely used in making Paleo keto bread. This ingredient gives the bread some chewiness and makes it sturdier. Even without it, other ingredients can still help achieve these.

2. Avocado Bacon and Egg

Literally, this looks like you're filling an avocado with egg. This delicious food will make a good breakfast and help achieve the belly-fat-burning goal. This recipe is meant to be good enough for two servings.

Ingredients:

- 1 medium-size avocado
- 2 eggs
- 1 piece of cooked and crumbled bacon
- Salt to taste
- 1 tablespoon of low-fat cheese

Instructions:

- Preheat the oven to reach temperature of 425 degrees Fahrenheit
- Cut the avocado into two equal halves and remove the pit.
- Scoop out some of the avocado with a spoon so you can have enough space to accommodate the egg. Place the avocado on a muffin pan to achieve stability while you're cooking.
- Break the eggs and pour in the cavities you already made in the avocado.
- Sprinkle salt and some cheese on it and cook for about 15 minutes
- Serve it while it is warm.

3. Grain-free hemp heart keto porridge

This ketogenic diet is made with seeds and nuts. It is free of sugar, diary, yeast and gluten. A great low-carb keto diet meal for every morning!

Ingredients:

- 1 tablespoon of chia seeds
- 2 tablespoons of freshly-ground flax seeds
- A cup of non-diary milk
- 5 drops of stevia that is free of alcohol
- ½ teaspoon of well-ground cinnamon
- ¼ cup of ground almond
- ½ teaspoon of vanilla extract
- ½ cup of Manitoba Harvest Hemp Hearts

Toppings:

- 3 fresh Brazil nuts
- A tablespoon of Manitoba Harvest Hemp Hearts

Instructions:

- Mix all the ingredients together, except the extras and ground almond in a small saucepan.
- Stir until they are well mixed together.

- Place in an oven or equivalent heating system until it begins to boil lightly.
- Leave it uncovered while the heating process is on-going.
- When it begins to bubble, stir and leave for another 2 minutes.
- Remove the heat and stir it in the already-crushed almonds.
- Turn it in a bowl, add the toppings and eat before it gets cold.

4. Low-carb sausage egg muffins

These low-carb egg muffins are the real grab-and-go breakfast that will leave your stomach filled for the day.

Ingredients:

- Half of a 16-oz roll of mild sausage for breakfast
- ¼ medium-size finely-chopped yellow onion, preferably about 3 teaspoons
- ½ teaspoon of crushed red pepper
- Six fresh eggs
- ½ teaspoon of paprika
- Pinch of salt to taste
- ¼ teaspoon of black pepper
- ¼ filled cup of milk
- Either of Mexican blend cheese or shredded cheddar

Instructions:

- Preheat the oven to hit a temperature of 400 degrees
- Spray each of the tins in a 12-cup muffin pan with standard cooking spray
- Cook the mixture of sausage, crushed pepper and chopped onion in a large skillet over heat.

- Leave until the sausage is cooked.
- Divide the cooked sausage mixture evenly amongst the 12 cups on the muffin pan.
- In a separate bowl, whisk together eggs, salt, milk, paprika and black pepper until they are bubbly and well mixed.
- Pour the mixture evenly on each of the muffin tin, just exactly on top of your sausage.
- Put the shredded cheese (or Mexican blend cheese) on each muffin.
- Bake it for 20 minutes over a 400-degree temperate.
- Allow the finished egg muffins to cool for a few minutes, and use a butter knife to loosen the edges on order to pop them out of the tins neatly.

5. Berry and whipped cream keto pancakes

A taste of this keto cottage cheese pancake is so incredible that you will not think of going back to your regular flapjacks. The berry that sits on top of it gives it the natural sweetness you crave.

Ingredients:

- 4 fresh eggs
- 7 oz cottage cheese
- 2 oz coconut oil or butter
- 1 tablespoon of ground psyllium husk powder

Toppings:

- ½ filled cup of fresh berries (strawberry, raspberry or blueberry)
- 1 cup filled with whipping cream

Instructions:

- Mix the eggs, psyllium husk powder and cottage cheese in a small bowl.
- Allow the mixture sit for about 8 minutes so that it can thicken up.
- Add some heat to your coconut oil or butter in a skillet that doesn't stick.

- Fry the pancakes for 3 minutes on a medium heat supply.
- Ensure the pancakes are not too big so that they don't become too hard to flip.
- In a separate bowl, whip the cream until soft peaks are formed.
- Serve the finished pancakes with the berry you have chosen and whipped cream.

6. Keto breakfast smoothie

There are keto dieters that really love the idea of gulping some smoothies down their throats every morning and still want to remain on keto. Here's the simplest keto smoothie for you.

Ingredients:

- ½ cup canned coconut milk
- 4 freshly-chopped strawberries
- ½ cup almond milk
- ¼ cup coconut yogurt
- ½ teaspoon of stevia
- ½ scoop of low-carb protein powder

Instructions:

- Assemble all the ingredients and blend in a food processor
- Pour into a cup
- Gulp or sip to your satisfaction

7. Low-carb keto hot pockets

There pockets are delicious and good enough to keep as part of your ketogenic lifestyle. These pockets are very simple to prepare and offers the qualities of every keto diet.

Ingredients:

- ¾ cup of shredded Mozzarella
- 2 fresh eggs
- 2 tablespoons of unsalted butter
- 3 slices OG cooked bacon
- ⅓ cup of almond flour

Instructions:

- Melt the mozzarella in a pan, add the almond flour to it and stir well.
- Roll out the dough between two parchment paper sheets
- Scramble the two eggs and mix with butter
- Lay the scrambled eggs along the center of your dough with bacon slices.
- Roll together and fold the dough
- Use a fork to make some holes on the dough surface to allow steam puff out during baking.

- Put in an oven for 20 minutes under a 400-degree Fahrenheit temperature until it turns golden brown and firm when touched.
- Serve and enjoy while it is hot.

8. Cheesy sausage puffs

These puffs are pretty easy and quick to prepare. With the instructions below and ingredients listed below, you can easily make some low-carb keto snacks.

Ingredients:

- 1 pound of hot Jimmy Dean sausage
- 2 cups of fresh shredded cheddar cheese
- 4 fresh eggs
- ⅓ cup of coconut flour
- ¼ tablespoon of salt
- ¼ tablespoon of baking powder
- 4½ tablespoon of melted butter
- 2 tablespoons of sour cream (or preferably softened cream cheese)

Instructions:

- Preheat the oven to reach 375-degree temperature.
- Melt the butter and allow to cool.
- Like a large baking sheet with parchment paper.
- Make the sausage turn brown and chop with knife into small chunks. Remove excess grease or pat it with paper towel until it dries.

- Whisk the melted butter, sour cream, eggs, salt and garlic (optional) in a medium-size container.
- Add baking powder and coconut flour, whisk them together until you achieve a well-combined result.
- Stir this in the browned sausage you prepared earlier and cheese.
- Roll batter into 1-inch balls on the baking sheet you had lined earlier.
- Put in oven and bake for 15 minutes until you notice it is getting slightly brown.
- Serve and enjoy the snacks while it is hot.

9. Chocolate coconut butter keto breakie

There's obviously no better way to start your day than with something that is as nutritious as this chocolate keto. In just five minutes, you can prepare this simple keto syrup.

Ingredients:

- 240ml diary-free milk
- 40g of chia seeds
- 3 tablespoons of cocoa powder
- 1 tablespoon of vanilla extract
- 2 tablespoons of either honey, agave or maple syrup sweetener.

Topping:

- Sliced banana or chocolate chips

Instructions:

- Combine all the ingredients in a large container and whisk until they are well-combined.
- Cover the container and put in refrigerator for 3 hours. You may as well refrigerate it overnight.
- Add your favorite topping and enjoy every sip.

10. High-fat low-carb berry chia pudding with coconut milk

This completely-creamy and sugar-free delicious breakie will give you the real satisfaction. It contains high fats and low carbs, hence, a good way to go ketogenic!

Ingredients:

- 1 large unsweetened shredded coconut
- 3 cups of water
- 3 cups of fresh coconut milk
- 2 cups of frozen or fresh berries
- 2 pinches of sea salt to balance flavor and taste
- Stevia or other sweetener of your choice
- 5-7 tablespoons of chia seeds
- 2 tablespoons of MCT oil
- 2 tablespoons of protein powder

Topping:

- Strawberries, blueberries or toasted coconut

Instructions:

- First prepare a fresh coconut milk by adding the shredded coconut to a blender and mix until it is finely ground. Add a cup of water and blend for a minute. Add another two cups of water to the blending coconut until the milk becomes creamy.

- Mix the berries with the coconut milk, MCT oil and protein powder.
- Add stevia and two pinches offer salt for sweetness and flavor balance.
- Pour the berry coconut milk in a bowl and stir with your chia seeds.
- Refrigerate it overnight so that you have it thick.
- Add your topping of choice right before you serve.

11. Keto Mug Lasagna

Lasagna is good for lunch, check out the simple instructions and make a delicious one for yourself.

Ingredients:

- 65g of zucchini
- 3 tablespoons of Rao's marinara
- 2 tablespoons whole milk of ricotta
- 3 ounces whole milk of mozzarella

Instructions:

- Use a sharp knife to slice the zucchini so thin like papers.
- Add one tablespoon of marinara at the bottom of your dish.
- Layer out on the sliced zucchini.
- Use a knife to spread out one tablespoon of ricotta.
- Put another tablespoon of marinara.
- Layer on another layer of zucchini, another tablespoon of ricotta, the remaining zucchini and the last teaspoon of Rao's marinara.
- Top the meal with mozzarella.
- Put in a microwave for 4 minutes under moderate temperature. You may sprinkle a little Parmesan cheese or some Oregano on it.

12. Grain-free keto chicken sandwich

Sandwiches are good lunch options. A delish chicken sandwich is remarkably easy to make. In just 30 minutes (or less), your lunch meal is ready!

Ingredients

For the chicken:

- 200g sliced chicken pieces
- 1 whisked egg
- 3g of garlic powder
- 5g of paprika
- Pinch of salt and dash of pepper
- Olive or avocado oil to fry the chicken

For the grain-free bread:

- 35g of almond of almond
- 1g of Italian seasoning
- 1g of baking powder
- 1g of salt
- 1 whisked egg
- 35ml of melted butter

Served with:

- Paleo mayo, mustard and romaine lettuce

Instructions

- Preheat the oven to reach 400F
- Put all the bread ingredients in a mug and mix thoroughly well
- Put the mug into microwave for 1½ minutes
- Allow the bread to cool down for some minutes and pop it out of the mug neatly with a clean knife and slice into 4.
- Cut the chicken breast into thin slices that can sit comfortably sit in the mug.
- Mix the egg, paprika, garlic powder, salt and pepper together to make coating for the chicken.
- Drop two tablespoons of oil into a frying pan. Dip each sliced chicken into the egg mixture and transfer into the prepared frying pan. Fry until the chicken turns golden brown and completely cooked. Put the sliced chicken pieces in a plate.
- Put the already-made sandwich together with some Paleo mayo, mustard and romaine lettuce leaves.

13. Sugar-free low-carb crustless Quiche

Excess eggs at home can be turned into something nutritious and delicious in just few minutes. The crustless quiche meal is prepared with lots of promising ingredients

Ingredients:

- ¼ cup of chopped onion
- 6 medium-size eggs
- ½ cup of cooked chopped sausage
- ¼ tablespoon of black pepper
- ½ cup of chopped spinach
- 1 tablespoon of cooking oil
- ¼ cup of bell pepper
- ½ cup of mushroom

Instructions:

- Preheat the oven to hit a temperature of 350F.
- Beat the eggs and mix them thoroughly in a medium-size bowl.
- Add all the ingredients in the mixture and mix again.
- Grease your frying pan with some oil.
- Turn the mixture into pan.

- Put the pan gently in the oven and let it be in there for 45 minutes. When the middle is set, it shows it is ready to eat.
- Slice the finished quiche and serve

14. Low-carb Broccoli Mushroom Frittata

The broccoli mushroom frittata is an affordable meal you can enjoy as brunch on Sundays as well as dinner on any other day you feel like going meatless.

Ingredients:

- A dash of black pepper for saucy taste
- 2 tablespoons of olive oil
- 8 oz sliced white mushrooms
- 2 tablespoons of diced yellow onion
- 2 cups of freshly-chopped broccoli florets
- 8 fresh eggs
- 2 minced cloves garlic

Instructions:

- Preheat your oven to a 400-degree temperature
- Heat the olive oil over a medium supply of her at in a skillet until it begins to shimmer.
- Add mushrooms, onion, pepper and salt.
- Sauté the mixture and stir occasionally.
- Add broccoli and garlic and continue the occasional stirring until your broccoli turns bright green and crisp-tender for about 5 minutes.

- Whisk together the pepper, eggs, mustard and milk until they are blended well and frothy enough
- Keep sautéing the vegetables
- Turn the egg mixture over the vegetables into the skillet.
- Continue cooking the mixture over medium heat supply until you observe that the edges begin to set.
- Turn off the heat. Top the egg with the shredded cheddar evenly, then take the skillet into the oven and allow for 15 minutes at 400 degrees. Broil to brown for a few minutes, and let the temperature cool down before you begin to slice the frittata.

15. Low-carb crack slaw egg roll

This is one of the easiest ketogenic meals for dinner

Ingredients:

- 4 tablespoons of avocado oil
- 4 minced cloves garlic
- 1 teaspoon of sea salt to taste
- ¼ cup of green onions
- 3 tablespoons of freshly-grated ginger
- 4 cups of shredded coleslaw mix
- 2 tablespoons of toasted sesame oil
- ¼ tablespoon of black pepper
- 1 lb of ground beef
- ¼ cup of coconut amino

Instructions:

- Heat the avocado oil on a medium heat supply in a large sauté pan. Add the ginger and garlic and sauté for another minute.
- Add the ground beef and season with salt
- Cook for about 8 minutes (or preferably till it gets browned).
- Add the coconut aminos and coleslaw mix and stir them together to coat, under a reduced heat supply. Cover it and cook for

the next 5 minutes until the cabbage becomes tender.

- Remove the heat and stir in the green oil and toasted sesame.

16. Low-carb baked turkey broccoli

The idea behind using turkey to make a broccoli sausage gives a delicious combination. For every keto dieter, this is a perfect meal for dinner.

Ingredients:

- ½ tablespoon of olive oil
- 4 oz offer shredded cheddar cheese
- ¼ of a medium-size diced yellow onion
- ½ tablespoon of chili powder
- 2 cups of freshly-chopped broccoli florets
- 4 oz of softened cream cheese
- 2 chopped cloves garlic
- 1 cup of chopped, cooked turkey
- ⅓ cup of salsa Verde
- Juice of ¼ of a small lime
- ½ tablespoon of cumin
- ½ tablespoon of smoked paprika
- Pinch of sea salt to taste
- 3 low-carb wraps
- ½ tablespoon of crushed pepper
- Olive oil cooking spray

Instructions:

- Take a chilled cream cheese from the refrigerator and allow to soften for about 20 minutes before you embark on cooking.
- Preheat your oven to hit 425 degrees.
- Line the baking sheet with foil and spray with the cooking spray oil.
- Heat the olive oil in a skillet until it begins to shimmer. Add onion, broccoli florets, crushed pepper and garlic. Sauté together for five minutes (until the broccoli turns bright green and somewhat tender).
- Add the chopped turkey to the cream cheese, cheddar cheese, salsa Verde, Chili powder, smoked paprika and cumin in a big bowl. Stir all the ingredients in the broccoli once the meal is cooked.
- Cut each of the low carbs in half and add a spoonful of the turkey mixture to the center of each wrap.
- Roll the wraps up and make them tight enough.
- Place them on the baking sheet.
- Spray the taquitos with cooking spray oil and sprinkle salt over it.

- Bake in oven regulated at 425 degree for an average of 15 minutes (preferably till it turns brown)
- Serve your meal with sour cream and/or salsa.

17. Low-carb pressure cooker zuppa Toscana

Many keto dieters do not like the idea of eating heavy dinner, hence a need to switch to his delicious meal

Ingredients:

- 1 chopped onion
- 2 tablespoons of pepper
- 1½ cup of coconut milk
- 2 tablespoons of cayenne
- 1 lb of Italian sausage
- 4 cups of chicken broth
- 1 head of chopped cauliflower without stem
- 2 cups fresh of kale
- 3 cloves of garlic
- 1 tablespoon of salt

Topping:

- Parmesan

Instructions:

- Turn the pressure cooker to SEAR and brown the Italian sausage
- Remove the drain and add the chopped onion and cook until it is soft.
- Add garlic and cook for the next 3 minutes.

- Add the seasonings, chicken broth, cauliflower and sausage.
- Close the lid and cook for another 5 minutes.
- Add kale and coconut milk until the kale wilts. Ensure the cauliflower doesn't break.
- Once the kale is wilted, serve and top with Parmesan and enjoy the delicacy.

18. Instant Pot Spaghetti Squash with Meat Sauce.

If you have an Instant Pot, preparing this spaghetti squash will be much easier and more enjoyable, all you need to do is follow these simple instructions.

Ingredients:

- 1 diced green pepper
- 1 lb. of fresh sausage
- 1 large spaghetti squash
- 1 small diced onion
- 25 oz. organic pasta sauce
- 4 oz. of fresh, pressed garlic
- 8 oz. often freshly-sliced mushroom

Instructions:

- Put the inner pot in the Instant pot
- Put fresh sausage in the inner pot and sauce.
- Toss the sausage occasionally until it gets browned.
- Drain after it is browned.
- Turn in the pot and add the vegetables.
- Cook and stir continuously for 5 minutes.
- After the veggies have become somewhat soft, add the pasta sauce and continue stirring for a few minutes.

- Mix spaghetti squash with the sauce or rather top it with the meat sauce.

19. Ham & Cheese Quiche Cups

Ham is naturally simple and easy to cook, plus it's a good keto option.

Ingredients:

- 1 cup of grated cheddar cheese
- 6 fresh eggs
- 1 tablespoon of salt
- 1 cup of cubed ham
- 1 big green onion
- 1 small diced tomato
- ½ tablespoon of pepper

Instructions

- Preheat your oven to hit a temperature of 400 degrees.
- While every other thing is being prepared, spray a large muffin tin with non-stick spray. Put in oven afterwards.
- Beat the eggs with the edge of a knife and mix thoroughly in a medium-size bowl.
- Add the onion, salt, ham, tomato, pepper and half of the cheese to the bowl to of egg and mix the ingredients together thoroughly.
- Top the 12 cups with the left-over cheese.
- Bake it in the oven for about 16 minutes until it is thoroughly cooked.

20. Zucchini Pizza with Double Cheese

Ingredients:

- 200g of pepperoni
- 1 large zucchini
- ⅓ cup of homemade sugar-free pizza sauce
- Pepper and salt to taste
- ⅓ grated mozzarella cheese
- ⅓ grated cheddar cheese
- ⅛ teaspoon of ground Sage
- ⅛ teaspoon of dried basil
- Fresh minced cilantro

Instructions:

- Preheat your oven to reach 350 degrees temperature.
- Wash the zucchini properly and thoroughly. Leave the skin or peel from top to end (depending on how you'll like it to be).
- Slice the zucchini into about ¼ inch per slice.
- Season your sliced zucchini ground black pepper, basil and sage. Take it to the oven and allow it to be in there for next 4-5 minutes.
- Add ½ teaspoon of pizza sauce on each sliced zucchini. Top each slice of zucchini

withpepperoni. Then, bake it for another 7 minutes or until the sides of pepperoni get browned.

- Withdraw from the oven and spill some cheese on top. Spill one side with mozzarella and the other side with cheddar. Top the mozzarella cheese side with a slice of black olives. Bake for 5 minutes or until cheese melts.
- Check occasionally to ensure the pepperoni is not sliding to the side and just slowly push back to the center with tongs or fork.
- Allow it cool and slowly transfer the meal to a platter.
- Add minced cilantro to the finished meal for garnishing

21. Mexican Chicken soup

Ingredients:

- 1½ pounds of boneless chicken thigh pieces
- 8 ounces of shredded Pepper Jack cheese or Monterey
- 15.5 ounces of chunky salsa
- 15 ounces of chicken bone broth

Instructions:

- Put the chicken pieces at the bottom of a crock pot.
- Add all other ingredients listed above.
- Cook on a medium heat supply for about 6 hours.
- Remove the shred chicken and chicken pieces, and return them to crock.
- Serve while it is hot.

22. Low-carb cauliflower Pizza crust

Ingredients:

- 1 medium-size cauliflower head
- 2 tablespoons of Italian Seasoning
- 1 fresh egg
- 1 tablespoon of dried Parsley
- Pepper and salt for sauciness and taste
- ⅓ cup of shredded Mozzarella Cheese
- 3 chopped Basil leaves
- ⅓ cup or shredded Parmesan Cheese
- 8 oz of shredded Mozzarella cheese
- ¼ cup of tomato sauce

Instructions:

- Preheat your oven to hit 400 Fahrenheit temperature.
- Spray a cookie sheet with cooking oil and line the oven.
- Cut your cauliflower into florets, and blend together in food processor until it looks like rice.
- Turn the processed cauliflower rice in a bowl and microwave it for about 3 minutes.
- Let it cool and pour inside a thin dish towel.

- Wrap the cauliflower in dish towel, twist and wring it hard enough to get rid of all liquid present in the cauliflower so that the crust can come together.
- Turn the cauliflower inside a bowl with all other ingredients and mix thoroughly with hands. Form into a ball and plan on top of the prepared sheet in the oven and bake for 8 minutes (preferably till it beings to turn golden)
- Take it from the oven and add any topping of your choice.
- Put back in the oven and observe till the cheese melts
- Remove from the oven, slice into pieces and serve!

23. Baked Salmon with creamy garlic yoghurt

Ingredients:

- 4 salmon fillets
- ¼ tablespoon of salt
- 2 tablespoons of chili powder
- ¼ lemon, squeezed
- 5 oz of plain Greek yogurt
- 2 minced garlic cloves
- ½ bunch of finely-chopped fresh dill

Instructions:

- Preheat the oven to hit a temperature of 425 Fahrenheit.
- Line the oven with a cookie sheet with a parchment paper.
- Rub salt and chili powder on the surface of the salmon fillets.
- Place salmon on a neat baking sheet, put inside oven and bake for 13 minutes.
- In a big bowl, make a creamy sauce by combining the Greek yogurt, fresh lemon juice, fresh dill and minced garlic.
- Remove the baked salmon from the oven, turn on a big plate and top with the creamy sauce.

24. Low-carb creamy peanut butter chocolate fudge

Ingredients:

- 4 squares of unsweetened baking chocolate
- 1 teaspoon of vanilla
- 1 filled cup of all-natural peanut butter
- ½ cup of Truvia sweetener
- ½ cup of fat-free half-and-half

Instructions:

- Melt the chocolate over medium supply of heat.
- Mix the melted chocolate with half-and-half and sweetener, then stir until it dissolves totally.
- After you have dissolved the chocolate, take it off the heater, stir the vanilla and peanut butter together and mix them thoroughly until it is smooth.
- Place the fudge in a square container and smoothen with spatula and allow to cool.
- When it's cool, cut your fudge into pieces.
- Cover and store them in a refrigerator.

25. Low-carb chocolate cheesecake dessert

Ingredients:

- 4 oz of softened cream cheese
- ¾ cup of heavy cream
- ½ cup of toasted and unsweetened coconut
- ⅛ teaspoon of vanilla cream liquid stevia
- 5 tablespoons of swerve sweetener
- 3 tablespoons of unsweetened cocoa
- ½ cup of roasted and chopped pecans.

Instructions

- Mix Swerve, cream cheese and heavy cream in a big bowl and best together until well mixed.
- Add all other ingredients (except pecans and coconut) and beat together until it becomes creamy.
- Put the creamy mixture in a refrigerator for about an hour so it becomes hard a bit.
- In a dry skillet, toast the unsweetened coconut. Put the pecans in another skillet and toast.
- Allow it to cool and put in bowls and set them aside.

- Take the cream cheese mixture from the refrigerator and scoop out a spoonful and add in the coconut mixture. Roll them mixture into a smooth ball and put in a clean and dry plate. Serve!

26. Low-carb Chicken cordon bleu casserole

Ingredients:

- 1 head of Cauliflower florets
- ¼ cup of avocado oil
- Black pepper and sea salt
- ⅓ cup of heavy cream
- 1½ lb. of shredded chicken breast
- ½ cup of sour cream
- 2 cloves of minced garlic
- 2 tablespoons of Dijon mustard
- ¼ cup of pork rinds
- 12 oz. of chopped Ham
- 2 cups of shredded Swiss cheese
- Chopped chives

Instructions:

- Preheat your oven to reach 450 degrees Fahrenheit.
- Toss the cauliflower and oil in a medium-size bowl
- Add black pepper and salt.
- Put the cauliflower on a baking sheet and roast in the oven until you observe golden brown on the edges.

- Stir the mustard, cream, half of the shredded cheese, garlic and sour cream in a big bowl, together with ham and chicken.
- Take the cauliflower out of the oven and lower the oven temperature to about 400 degrees and stir the cauliflower in the bowl.
- Take the casserole mixture and put in a casserole dish. Top it with the remaining 1 cup of shredded Swiss cheese. You may sprinkle crushed pork rinds.
- Take to oven and bake until the cheese turns golden and melts, and the casserole is becomes bubbly.
- You may now garnish it with some fresh chives.

27. Instant Pot Chicken tika masala

Ingredients:

- 2 lbs of boneless skinless Chicken breast
- Coconut oil
- 2 of 14 oz cans diced tomatoes
- Diced sweet onion
- 1 tablespoon of plain almond butter
- Crushed garlic
- Half to one cup of unsweetened coconut milk
- Crushed garlic
- 1 small diced seeded jalapeño
- Salt, chili powder and pepper
- 1 tablespoon of peeled, diced ginger
- ½ tablespoon of lime
- Chard, mushroom or any vegetable of your choice
- Fresh Cilantro

Instructions:

- Regulate your Instant Pot to "Sauté" and pour in coconut oil. Allow it melt.
- Add chopped onions and stir until it is softened
- Add chili powder and other spices, then stir.

- Add your diced ginger, garlic, chopped jalapeño, the two tomato cans and any optional vegetable you have chosen.
- Add chicken and stir together to get the chicken covered with the spices.
- Seal the Instant Pot lid tightly and press the Manual button. Set the timer to 15 minutes.
- After 15 minutes is up, open the valve. After the steam might have escaped, escaped, take off the lid.
- Take out the chicken from the pot and put in a bowl. Place it aside.
- Put the mixture in a food processor, add lime juice, coconut milk and almond butter. Blend together until it is smooth. Put this onto the chicken and stir evenly.
- Put this on a bed of Cauliflower rice.
- Put some chopped cilantro on it for garnish.
- Serve and enjoy!

28. Garlic Shrimp Zoodles

Ingredients:

- 2 medium-size of zucchini
- 1 tablespoon of olive oil
- ¾ pounds of medium peeled and deveined shrimp
- Flakes of red pepper
- Zest and juice of a lemon
- 3-4 cloves of minced garlic
- Pepper & salt to taste
- Fresh chopped parsley

Instructions:

- Make the zucchini into medium-size spirals and put aside.
- Put a skillet on medium heat, add lemon juice, olive oil and zest. Once the pan is warm, put in the shrimp.
- Cook the shrimp and turn the other side at the end of 1 minute.
- Add pepper flakes and garlic. Cook this for another minute, and stir often.
- Now, put the zucchini noodles and stir constantly with tongs constantly for next two minutes until you notice they're warmed up and slightly cooked.

- Add your seasonings salt and sprinkle the chopped parsley on top.
- Serve while it's hot.

29. Low-carb curried riced cauliflower and shrimp

Ingredients:

- 1 bag of Green Giant Riced Cauliflower
- 1 chopped onion
- ½ chopped Red Pepper
- 2 tablespoons of chopped parsley
- 1 lb of peeled and deveined uncooked shrimp
- 2 cloves of minced garlic
- ¾ cup of low Sodium Chicken Stock
- 2 teaspoons of curry Powder
- 1 teaspoon of cumin
- 2 teaspoons of olive oil
- 1 teaspoon of smoked paprika
- Pepper and salt
- Juice from Half a Lime

Instructions:

- Put skillet on a medium heat supply, add the olive oil.
- Put the pepper, onion, salt and stir continuously until they are softened. Put garlic and cook for the next minute

- Add the whole bag of Green Giant Riced Cauliflower into the skillet and mix together with a spatula.
- Put curry, cumin and smoked paprika, and stir.
- Then add the chicken stock. Reduce the heat supply to medium-low.
- Add salt and pepper to the shrimp and them into the cauliflower rice.
- Cover it and cook for about three minutes. Do not allow the shrimp overcook.
- Remove the cover and add the parsley. Pour in the lime juice and stir continuously.
- Turn off the heat and serve!

30. Cloud bread

Ingredients:

- 3 divided large eggs
- ⅛ teaspoon cream of tartar
- 3 tablespoons of cream cheese/ ⅓ cup of light Greek yogurt

Instructions:

- Preheat your oven to 300 degrees Fahrenheit.
- Line pan with parchment paper.
- Mix cream of tartar with egg whites on high speed until you notice the formation of stiff peaks.
- Mix egg yolks & Greek yogurt (or cream cheese) in a large bowl until they are well combined. Pour in about 1 cup of the egg white mixture until they are well combined. Then, add the remaining egg whites and fold just until it is well-mixed.
- Now, on the prepared pan, divide the egg mixture into 6 portions equally.
- Spread the mixture until it is about ½ inch thick.
- Bake the mixture until it turns lightly browned.

- Afterwards, cool it in a wire rack for about 60 minutes.
- Put the baked mixture in a sealed container and refrigerate.

References

[1] C. de Duve, "The lysosome turns fifty," *Nat. Cell Biol.*, vol. 7, p. 847, Sep. 2005.

[2] S. Cohen, "Lysosomes Ciba Foundation Symposium," *Postgrad. Med. J.*, vol. 40, no. 467, p. 557, Sep. 1964.

[3] B. Levine and G. Kroemer, "Autophagy in the Pathogenesis of Disease," *Cell*, vol. 132, no. 1, p. 27, 2008.

[4] N. Mizushima, "Autophagy: process and function," *Genes Dev.*, vol. 21, pp. 2861–2873, 2007.

[5] W. Li, J. Li, and J. Bao, "Microautophagy: lesser-known self-eating.," *Cell. Mol. Life Sci.*, vol. 69, no. 7, pp. 1125–36, Apr. 2012.

[6] S. Kaushik and A. M. Cuervo, "Chaperone-mediated autophagy: a unique way to enter the lysosome world.," *Trends Cell Biol.*, vol. 22, no. 8, pp. 407–17, Aug. 2012.

[7] M. A. Hayat, "Introduction to Autophagy," *Autophagy Cancer, Other Pathol. Inflammation, Immunity, Infect. Aging*, 2015.

[8] K. Yoshimoto *et al.*, "Processing of ATG8s,

"

Ubiquitin-Like Proteins, and Their Deconjugation by ATG4s Are Essential for Plant Autophagy," *Plant Cell*, vol. 16, no. 11, pp. 2967 LP – 2983, Nov. 2004.

[9]   J. J. Lum, R. J. DeBerardinis, and C. B. Thompson, "Autophagy in metazoans: cell survival in the land of plenty.," *Nat. Rev. Mol. Cell Biol.*, vol. 6, no. 6, pp. 439–48, Jun. 2005.

[10]   A. Sotthibundhu *et al.*, "Rapamycin regulates autophagy and cell adhesion in induced pluripotent stem cells.," *Stem Cell Res. Ther.*, vol. 7, no. 1, p. 166, 2016.

[11]   H. Nakatogawa, Y. Ichimura, and Y. Ohsumi, "Atg8, a ubiquitin-like protein required for autophagosome formation, mediates membrane tethering and hemifusion," *Cell*, vol. 130, no. 1, pp. 165–178, 2007.

[12]   D. J. Klionsky, A. M. Cuervo, and P. O. Seglen, "Methods for monitoring autophagy from yeast to human," *Autophagy*, vol. 3, no. 3, pp. 181–206, 2007.

[13]   C. Sagné *et al.*, "Identification and characterization of a lysosomal transporter for small neutral amino acids."

[14]   P.-Y. Ke, "The Multifaceted Roles of

Autophagy in Flavivirus-Host Interactions," *Int. J. Mol. Sci.*, vol. 19, no. 12, p. 3940, Dec. 2018.

[15] U. Pfeifer and P. Strauss, "Autophagic vacuoles in heart muscle and liver. A comparative morphometric study including circadian variations in meal-fed rats.," *J. Mol. Cell. Cardiol.*, vol. 13, no. 1, pp. 37–49, Jan. 1981.

[16] R. McCormick and A. Vasilaki, "Age-related changes in skeletal muscle: changes to life-style as a therapy," *Biogerontology*, vol. 19, no. 6, pp. 519–536, Dec. 2018.

[17] U. Pfeifer and M. Warmuth-Metz, "Inhibition by insulin of cellular autophagy in proximal tubular cells of rat kidney," *Am. J. Physiol. Metab.*, vol. 244, no. 2, pp. E109–E114, Feb. 1983.

[18] N. Mizushima and D. J. Klionsky, "Protein turnover via autophagy: implications for metabolism.," *Annu. Rev. Nutr.*, vol. 27, pp. 19–40, 2007.

[19] X. Qu *et al.*, "Autophagy gene-dependent clearance of apoptotic cells during embryonic development.," *Cell*, vol. 128, no. 5, pp. 931–46, Mar. 2007.

[20] J. J. Lum *et al.*, "Growth factor regulation of autophagy and cell survival in the absence of apoptosis.," *Cell*, vol. 120, no. 2, pp. 237–48, Jan. 2005.

[21] J. J. Lum *et al.*, "Growth factor regulation of autophagy and cell survival in the absence of apoptosis.," *Cell*, vol. 120, no. 2, pp. 237–48, Jan. 2005.

[22] A. Kuma *et al.*, "The role of autophagy during the early neonatal starvation period.," *Nature*, vol. 432, no. 7020, pp. 1032–6, Dec. 2004.

[23] Y. T. Kwon and A. Ciechanover, "The Ubiquitin Code in the Ubiquitin-Proteasome System and Autophagy," *Trends Biochem. Sci.*, vol. 42, no. 11, pp. 873–886, Nov. 2017.

[24] Y. Zhang, X. Chen, Y. Zhao, M. Ponnusamy, and Y. Liu, "The role of ubiquitin proteasomal system and autophagy-lysosome pathway in Alzheimer's disease," *Rev. Neurosci.*, vol. 28, no. 8, pp. 861–868, Nov. 2017.

[25] I. Kim, S. Rodriguez-Enriquez, and J. J. Lemasters, "Selective degradation of mitochondria by mitophagy.," *Arch. Biochem. Biophys.*, vol. 462, no. 2, pp. 245–53, Jun. 2007.

[26] N. Mizushima and D. J. Klionsky, "Protein turnover via autophagy: implications for metabolism.," *Annu. Rev. Nutr.*, vol. 27, pp. 19–40, 2007.

[27] J. M. Bravo-San Pedro, G. Kroemer, and L. Galluzzi, "Autophagy and Mitophagy in Cardiovascular Disease," *Circ. Res.*, vol. 120, no. 11, pp. 1812–1824, May 2017.

[28] E. White, J. M. Mehnert, and C. S. Chan, "Autophagy, Metabolism, and Cancer," *Clin. Cancer Res.*, vol. 21, no. 22, pp. 5037–5046, Nov. 2015.

[29] V. V. Eapen *et al.*, "A pathway of targeted autophagy is induced by DNA damage in budding yeast," *Proc. Natl. Acad. Sci.*, vol. 114, no. 7, pp. E1158–E1167, Feb. 2017.

[30] L. Gomes, C. Menck, and G. Leandro, "Autophagy Roles in the Modulation of DNA Repair Pathways," *Int. J. Mol. Sci.*, vol. 18, no. 11, p. 2351, Nov. 2017.

[31] S. Jin and E. White, "Role of autophagy in cancer: management of metabolic stress.," *Autophagy*, vol. 3, no. 1, pp. 28–31, 2007.

[32] U. C. Anozie and P. Dalhaimer, "Molecular links among non-biodegradable nanoparticles,

reactive oxygen species, and autophagy," *Adv. Drug Deliv. Rev.*, vol. 122, pp. 65–73, Dec. 2017.

[33] Y.-F. Chen *et al.*, "The roles of reactive oxygen species (ROS) and autophagy in the survival and death of leukemia cells," *Crit. Rev. Oncol. Hematol.*, vol. 112, pp. 21–30, Apr. 2017.

[34] B. Albert, A. Johnson, J. Lweis, and E. Al., *Molecular Biology of the Cell*, 4th ed. New York: Garland Science, 2002.

[35] L. F. Díaz, M. Chiong, A. Quest, S. Lavandero, and A. Stutzin, "Mechanisms of cell death: molecular insights and therapeutic perspectives," *Cell Death Differ.*, vol. 12, pp. 1449–1456, 2005.

[36] K. Wang, "Autophagy and apoptosis in liver injury.," *Cell Cycle*, vol. 14, no. 11, pp. 1631–42, 2015.

[37] L. F. Díaz, M. Chiong, A. Quest, S. Lavandero, and A. Stutzin, "Mechanisms of cell death: molecular insights and therapeutic perspectives," *Cell Death Differ.*, vol. 12, pp. 1449–1456, 2005.

[38] S. Patschan *et al.*, "Lipid mediators of

autophagy in stress-induced premature senescence of endothelial cells," *Am. J. Physiol. Circ. Physiol.*, vol. 294, no. 3, pp. H1119–H1129, Mar. 2008.

[39] E. Bejarano, A. Yuste, B. Patel, R. F. Stout Jr, D. C. Spray, and A. M. Cuervo, "Connexins modulate autophagosome biogenesis," *Nat. Cell Biol.*, vol. 16, no. 5, pp. 401–414, May 2014.

[40] G. N. DeMartino, "Thematic Minireview Series - autophagy.," *J. Biol. Chem.*, 2018.

[41] S. Luo and D. C. Rubinsztein, "Apoptosis blocks Beclin 1-dependent autophagosome synthesis: an effect rescued by Bcl-xL.," *Cell Death Differ.*, vol. 17, no. 2, pp. 268–77, Feb. 2010.

[42] C. Gordy and Y.-W. He, "The crosstalk between autophagy and apoptosis: where does this lead?," *Protein Cell*, vol. 3, no. 1, pp. 17–27, Jan. 2012.

[43] W. Hou, J. Han, C. Lu, L. A. Goldstein, and H. Rabinowich, "Autophagic degradation of active caspase-8: a crosstalk mechanism between autophagy and apoptosis.," *Autophagy*, vol. 6, no. 7, pp. 891–900, Oct. 2010.

[44]   S. Ghavami *et al.*, "Autophagy and apoptosis dysfunction in neurodegenerative disorders," *Prog. Neurobiol.*, vol. 112, pp. 24–49, Jan. 2014.

[45]   A. V. Cybulsky, "Endoplasmic reticulum stress, the unfolded protein response and autophagy in kidney diseases," *Nat. Rev. Nephrol.*, vol. 13, no. 11, pp. 681–696, Oct. 2017.

[46]   D. C. Rubinsztein, J. E. Gestwicki, L. O. Murphy, and D. J. Klionsky, "Potential therapeutic applications of autophagy.," *Nat. Rev. Drug Discov.*, vol. 6, no. 4, pp. 304–12, Apr. 2007.

[47]   D. C. Rubinsztein, "The roles of intracellular protein-degradation pathways in neurodegeneration.," *Nature*, vol. 443, no. 7113, pp. 780–6, Oct. 2006.

[48]   M. García-Arencibia, W. E. Hochfeld, P. P. C. Toh, and D. C. Rubinsztein, "Autophagy, a guardian against neurodegeneration.," *Semin. Cell Dev. Biol.*, vol. 21, no. 7, pp. 691–8, Sep. 2010.

[49]   G. Šimić *et al.*, "Tau protein hyperphosphorylation and aggregation in Alzheimer's disease and other tauopathies,

and possible neuroprotective strategies," *Biomolecules*, vol. 6, no. 1, p. 6, 2016.

[50] R. A. Kern, R. Gonzalez, and I. Garitaonandia, "Use of neural cells derived from human pluripotent stem cells for the treatment of neurodegenerative diseases." US Patent App. 14/181,285, 07-Aug-2018.

[51] J. M. P. Ortiz and H. T. Orr, "Spinocerebellar Ataxia Type 1: Molecular Mechanisms of Neurodegeneration and Preclinical Studies," in *Polyglutamine Disorders*, Springer, 2018, pp. 135–145.

[52] S. Gelino *et al.*, "Intestinal autophagy improves healthspan and longevity in C. elegans during dietary restriction," *PLoS Genet.*, vol. 12, no. 7, p. e1006135, 2016.

[53] M. Moulis and C. Vindis, "Autophagy in Metabolic Age-Related Human Diseases.," *Cells*, vol. 7, no. 10, Sep. 2018.

[54] J. H. Ko, S.-O. Yoon, H. J. Lee, and J. Y. Oh, "Rapamycin regulates macrophage activation by inhibiting NLRP3 inflammasome-p38 MAPK-NFκB pathways in autophagy- and p62-dependent manners," *Oncotarget*, vol. 8, no. 25, pp. 40817–40831, Apr. 2017.

[55]   A. Relaño-Ginés *et al.*, "Lithium as a disease-modifying agent for prion diseases," *Transl. Psychiatry*, vol. 8, no. 1, p. 163, Aug. 2018.

[56]   R. Mathew *et al.*, "Autophagy suppresses tumorigenesis through elimination of p62.," *Cell*, vol. 137, no. 6, pp. 1062–75, Jun. 2009.

[57]   Z. J. Yang, C. E. Chee, S. Huang, and F. A. Sinicrope, "The role of autophagy in cancer: therapeutic implications.," *Mol. Cancer Ther.*, vol. 10, no. 9, pp. 1533–41, Sep. 2011.

[58]   W.-X. Ding *et al.*, "Autophagy reduces acute ethanol-induced hepatotoxicity and steatosis in mice.," *Gastroenterology*, vol. 139, no. 5, pp. 1740–52, Nov. 2010.

[59]   C.-W. Lin *et al.*, "Pharmacological promotion of autophagy alleviates steatosis and injury in alcoholic and non-alcoholic fatty liver conditions in mice.," *J. Hepatol.*, vol. 58, no. 5, pp. 993–9, May 2013.

[60]   W.-X. Ding *et al.*, "Autophagy reduces acute ethanol-induced hepatotoxicity and steatosis in mice.," *Gastroenterology*, vol. 139, no. 5, pp. 1740–52, Nov. 2010.

[61]   A. Takamura *et al.*, "Autophagy-deficient mice develop multiple liver tumors.," *Genes*

Dev., vol. 25, no. 8, pp. 795–800, Apr. 2011.

[62] S.-H. Lan *et al.*, "Autophagy suppresses tumorigenesis of hepatitis B virus-associated hepatocellular carcinoma through degradation of microRNA-224.," *Hepatology*, vol. 59, no. 2, pp. 505–17, Feb. 2014.

[63] S. Shrivastava, J. Bhanja Chowdhury, R. Steele, R. Ray, and R. B. Ray, "Hepatitis C virus upregulates Beclin1 for induction of autophagy and activates mTOR signaling.," *J. Virol.*, vol. 86, no. 16, pp. 8705–12, Aug. 2012.

[64] D. H. Perlmutter, "The role of autophagy in alpha-1-antitrypsin deficiency: a specific cellular response in genetic diseases associated with aggregation-prone proteins.," *Autophagy*, vol. 2, no. 4, pp. 258–63, 2006.

[65] T. Kamimoto *et al.*, "Intracellular inclusions containing mutant alpha1-antitrypsin Z are propagated in the absence of autophagic activity.," *J. Biol. Chem.*, vol. 281, no. 7, pp. 4467–76, Feb. 2006.

[66] T. Ueno and M. Komatsu, "Autophagy in the liver: functions in health and disease," *Nat. Rev. Gastroenterol. Hepatol.*, vol. 14, pp. 170–184, 2017.

[67] R. S. D'souza *et al.*, "Danon disease clinical features, evaluation, and management," *Circ. Hear. Fail.*, 2014.

[68] E. L. Eskelinen, "Roles of LAMP-1 and LAMP-2 in lysosome biogenesis and autophagy," *Molecular Aspects of Medicine*. 2006.

[69] J. Bolaños-Meade, L. Zhou, A. Hoke, A. Corse, G. Vogelsang, and K. R. Wagner, "Hydroxychloroquine causes severe vacuolar myopathy in a patient with chronic graft-versus-host disease.," *Am. J. Hematol.*, vol. 78, no. 4, pp. 306–9, Apr. 2005.

[70] M. Dasouki *et al.*, "Pompe disease: Literature review and case series," *Neurologic Clinics*. 2014.

[71] N. Raben *et al.*, "Suppression of autophagy permits successful enzyme replacement therapy in a lysosomal storage disorder - Murine Pompe disease," *Autophagy*, 2010.

[72] Z. Lu *et al.*, "The tumor suppressor gene ARHI regulates autophagy and tumor dormancy in human ovarian cancer cells.," *J. Clin. Invest.*, vol. 118, no. 12, pp. 3917–29, Dec. 2008.

[73] Z. Lu *et al.*, "The tumor suppressor gene ARHI regulates autophagy and tumor dormancy in human ovarian cancer cells.," *J. Clin. Invest.*, vol. 118, no. 12, pp. 3917–29, Dec. 2008.

[74] R. K. Amaravadi *et al.*, "Autophagy inhibition enhances therapy-induced apoptosis in a Myc-induced model of lymphoma.," *J. Clin. Invest.*, vol. 117, no. 2, pp. 326–36, Feb. 2007.

[75] M. C. Maiuri, E. Zalckvar, A. Kimchi, and G. Kroemer, "Self-eating and self-killing: crosstalk between autophagy and apoptosis.," *Nat. Rev. Mol. Cell Biol.*, vol. 8, no. 9, pp. 741–52, Sep. 2007.

[76] J. Han *et al.*, "Involvement of protective autophagy in TRAIL resistance of apoptosis-defective tumor cells.," *J. Biol. Chem.*, vol. 283, no. 28, pp. 19665–77, Jul. 2008.

[77] X. Li and Z. Fan, "The epidermal growth factor receptor antibody cetuximab induces autophagy in cancer cells by downregulating HIF-1alpha and Bcl-2 and activating the beclin 1/hVps34 complex.," *Cancer Res.*, vol. 70, no. 14, pp. 5942–52, Jul. 2010.

[78] J. J. Shacka, B. J. Klocke, and K. A. Roth, "Autophagy, bafilomycin and cell death: the

'a-B-cs' of plecomacrolide-induced neuroprotection.," *Autophagy*, vol. 2, no. 3, pp. 228–30.

[79] J. vB Hjelmborg *et al.*, "Genetic influence on human lifespan and longevity.," *Hum. Genet.*, vol. 119, no. 3, pp. 312–21, Apr. 2006.

[80] "Cannon, Walter Bradford (1871-1945) | Harvard Square Library." [Online]. Available: https://www.harvardsquarelibrary.org/biogra phies/walter-bradford-cannon-2/. [Accessed: 14-Mar-2019].

[81] B. Cannon, "Walter Bradford Cannon, M.D.: Reflections on the physician, the man, and his contributions.," *Gastrointest. Radiol.*, vol. 7, no. 1, pp. 1–6, 1982.

[82] Y. Riahi *et al.*, "Autophagy is a major regulator of beta cell insulin homeostasis.," *Diabetologia*, vol. 59, no. 7, pp. 1480–1491, 2016.

[83] S. Namkoong, C.-S. Cho, I. Semple, and J. H. Lee, "Autophagy Dysregulation and Obesity-Associated Pathologies.," *Mol. Cells*, vol. 41, no. 1, pp. 3–10, Jan. 2018.

[84] B. Jaishy and E. D. Abel, "Lipids, lysosomes, and autophagy.," *J. Lipid Res.*, vol. 57, no. 9,

pp. 1619–35, 2016.

[85] G. R. Y. De Meyer, M. O. J. Grootaert, C. F. Michiels, A. Kurdi, D. M. Schrijvers, and W. Martinet, "Autophagy in vascular disease.," *Circ. Res.*, vol. 116, no. 3, pp. 468–79, Jan. 2015.

[86] N. Martinez-Lopez, D. Athonvarangkul, and R. Singh, "Autophagy and Aging An Introduction to Autophagy HHS Public Access," *Adv Exp Med Biol*, vol. 847, pp. 73–87, 2015.

[87] M. Komatsu *et al.*, "Loss of autophagy in the central nervous system causes neurodegeneration in mice.," *Nature*, vol. 441, no. 7095, pp. 880–4, Jun. 2006.

[88] Y. Stroikin, H. Dalen, S. Lööf, and A. Terman, "Inhibition of autophagy with 3-methyladenine results in impaired turnover of lysosomes and accumulation of lipofuscin-like material.," *Eur. J. Cell Biol.*, vol. 83, no. 10, pp. 583–90, Oct. 2004.

[89] E. Masiero *et al.*, "Autophagy is required to maintain muscle mass.," *Cell Metab.*, vol. 10, no. 6, pp. 507–15, Dec. 2009.

[90] Z. Zhao *et al.*, "A dual role for UVRAG in

maintaining chromosomal stability independent of autophagy.," *Dev. Cell*, vol. 22, no. 5, pp. 1001–16, May 2012.

[91] A. Matsui, Y. Kamada, and A. Matsuura, "The role of autophagy in genome stability through suppression of abnormal mitosis under starvation.," *PLoS Genet.*, vol. 9, no. 1, p. e1003245, 2013.

[92] M. M. Lipinski *et al.*, "Genome-wide analysis reveals mechanisms modulating autophagy in normal brain aging and in Alzheimer's disease.," *Proc. Natl. Acad. Sci. U. S. A.*, vol. 107, no. 32, pp. 14164–9, Aug. 2010.

[93] A. Donati *et al.*, "Age-related changes in the autophagic proteolysis of rat isolated liver cells: effects of antiaging dietary restrictions.," *J. Gerontol. A. Biol. Sci. Med. Sci.*, vol. 56, no. 9, pp. B375-83, Sep. 2001.

[94] "Autophagy and aging."

[95] M. J. Czaja, "Autophagy in health and disease. 2. Regulation of lipid metabolism and storage by autophagy: pathophysiological implications.," *Am. J. Physiol. Cell Physiol.*, vol. 298, no. 5, pp. C973-8, May 2010.

[96] R. Singh *et al.*, "Autophagy regulates lipid

metabolism.," *Nature*, vol. 458, no. 7242, pp. 1131–5, Apr. 2009.

[97] R. Singh and A. M. Cuervo, "Lipophagy: Connecting Autophagy and Lipid Metabolism," *Int. J. Cell Biol.*, vol. 2012, pp. 1–12, 2012.

[98] A. Ost *et al.*, "Attenuated mTOR signaling and enhanced autophagy in adipocytes from obese patients with type 2 diabetes.," *Mol. Med.*, vol. 16, no. 7–8, pp. 235–46, 2010.

[99] "Obesity and overweight," *World Health Organization*, 2016. [Online]. Available: https://www.who.int/news-room/fact-sheets/detail/obesity-and-overweight. [Accessed: 19-Mar-2019].

[100] World Health Organization, "WHO - The top 10 causes of death," *24 Maggio*, 2018. .

[101] G. Fond, A. Macgregor, M. Leboyer, and A. Michalsen, "Fasting in mood disorders: neurobiology and effectiveness. A review of the literature.," *Psychiatry Res.*, vol. 209, no. 3, pp. 253–8, Oct. 2013.

[102] M. F. McCarty, J. J. DiNicolantonio, and J. H. O'Keefe, "Ketosis may promote brain macroautophagy by activating Sirt1 and

hypoxia-inducible factor-1," *Med. Hypotheses*, 2015.

[103] S. G. Hasselbalch, G. M. Knudsen, J. Jakobsen, L. P. Hageman, S. Holm, and O. B. Paulson, "Brain metabolism during short-term starvation in humans.," *J. Cereb. Blood Flow Metab.*, vol. 14, no. 1, pp. 125–31, Jan. 1994.

[104] G. F. Cahill, "Fuel metabolism in starvation.," *Annu. Rev. Nutr.*, vol. 26, pp. 1–22, 2006.

[105] E. Freemantle *et al.*, "Omega-3 fatty acids, energy substrates, and brain function during aging," *Prostaglandins, Leukot. Essent. Fat. Acids*, vol. 75, no. 3, pp. 213–220, Sep. 2006.

[106] J. M. Scott and P. A. Deuster, "Ketones and Human Performance.," *J. Spec. Oper. Med.*, vol. 17, no. 2, pp. 112–116.

[107] WHO, "CONSTITUTION OF THE WORLD HEALTH ORGANIZATION 1," Geneva, 2005.

[108] G. Canguihem, "What is health? The ability to adapt," 2009.

[109] N. Sartorius, "The Meanings of Health and its Promotion," *Croat Med J*, vol. 47, pp. 662–664, 2006.

[110] M. F. McCarty, J. J. DiNicolantonio, and J. H.

O'Keefe, "Ketosis may promote brain macroautophagy by activating Sirt1 and hypoxia-inducible factor-1.," *Med. Hypotheses*, vol. 85, no. 5, pp. 631–9, Nov. 2015.

[111] J. Leszek, E. Trypka, V. Tarasov, G. Ashraf, and G. Aliev, "Type 3 Diabetes Mellitus: A Novel Implication of Alzheimers Disease," *Curr. Top. Med. Chem.*, vol. 17, no. 12, pp. 1331–1335, Mar. 2017.

[112] S. C. Cunnane *et al.*, "Can Ketones Help Rescue Brain Fuel Supply in Later Life? Implications for Cognitive Health during Aging and the Treatment of Alzheimer's Disease.," *Front. Mol. Neurosci.*, vol. 9, p. 53, 2016.

[113] J. X. Yin *et al.*, "Ketones block amyloid entry and improve cognition in an Alzheimer's model," *Neurobiol. Aging*, vol. 39, pp. 25–37, Mar. 2016.

[114] S. T. Henderson, "Ketone bodies as a therapeutic for Alzheimer's disease," *Neurotherapeutics*, vol. 5, no. 3, pp. 470–480, Jul. 2008.

[115] T. A. Simeone, K. A. Simeone, C. E. Stafstrom, and J. M. Rho, "Do ketone bodies

mediate the anti-seizure effects of the ketogenic diet?," *Neuropharmacology*, vol. 133, pp. 233–241, 2018.

[116] T. Walczyk and J. Y. Wick, "The Ketogenic Diet: Making a Comeback.," *Consult. Pharm.*, vol. 32, no. 7, pp. 388–396, Jul. 2017.

[117] T. A. Simeone, K. A. Simeone, and J. M. Rho, "Ketone Bodies as Anti-Seizure Agents.," *Neurochem. Res.*, vol. 42, no. 7, pp. 2011–2018, Jul. 2017.

[118] M. A. McNally and A. L. Hartman, "Ketone bodies in epilepsy.," *J. Neurochem.*, vol. 121, no. 1, pp. 28–35, Apr. 2012.

[119] L. V Kalia and A. E. Lang, "Parkinson's disease.," *Lancet (London, England)*, vol. 386, no. 9996, pp. 896–912, Aug. 2015.

[120] J.-S. Park, R. L. Davis, and C. M. Sue, "Mitochondrial Dysfunction in Parkinson's Disease: New Mechanistic Insights and Therapeutic Perspectives," *Curr. Neurol. Neurosci. Rep.*, vol. 18, p. 21, 2018.

[121] M. C. L. Phillips, D. K. J. Murtagh, L. J. Gilbertson, F. J. S. Asztely, and C. D. P. Lynch, "Low-fat versus ketogenic diet in Parkinson's disease: A pilot randomized

controlled trial," *Mov. Disord.*, vol. 33, no. 8, pp. 1306–1314, Aug. 2018.

[122] D. M. Keller, "Ketogenic Diet Helps Nonmotor Symptoms in Parkinson's," 2018. [Online]. Available: https://www.medscape.com/viewarticle/9031 77. [Accessed: 21-Mar-2019].

[123] K. Tieu *et al.*, "D-beta-hydroxybutyrate rescues mitochondrial respiration and mitigates features of Parkinson disease.," *J. Clin. Invest.*, vol. 112, no. 6, pp. 892–901, Sep. 2003.

[124] K. J. Bough *et al.*, "Mitochondrial biogenesis in the anticonvulsant mechanism of the ketogenic diet.," *Ann. Neurol.*, vol. 60, no. 2, pp. 223–35, Aug. 2006.

[125] S. G. Jarrett, J. B. Milder, L.-P. Liang, and M. Patel, "The ketogenic diet increases mitochondrial glutathione levels," *J. Neurochem.*, vol. 106, no. 3, pp. 1044–1051, Aug. 2008.

[126] E. J. Gallagher and D. LeRoith, "Obesity and Diabetes: The Increased Risk of Cancer and Cancer-Related Mortality.," *Physiol. Rev.*, vol. 95, no. 3, pp. 727–48, Jul. 2015.

[127] G. Perseghin *et al.*, "Insulin resistance/hyperinsulinemia and cancer mortality: the Cremona study at the 15th year of follow-up.," *Acta Diabetol.*, vol. 49, no. 6, pp. 421–8, Dec. 2012.

[128] R. Madonna and R. De Caterina, "Atherogenesis and Diabetes: Focus on Insulin Resistance and Hyperinsulinemia," *Rev. Española Cardiol. (English Ed.*, vol. 65, no. 4, pp. 309–313, Apr. 2012.

[129] R. L. Veech, "The therapeutic implications of ketone bodies: the effects of ketone bodies in pathological conditions: ketosis, ketogenic diet, redox states, insulin resistance, and mitochondrial metabolism.," *Prostaglandins. Leukot. Essent. Fatty Acids*, vol. 70, no. 3, pp. 309–19, Mar. 2004.

[130] M. R. DiGruccio *et al.*, "Comprehensive alpha, beta and delta cell transcriptomes reveal that ghrelin selectively activates delta cells and promotes somatostatin release from pancreatic islets.," *Mol. Metab.*, vol. 5, no. 7, pp. 449–458, Jul. 2016.

[131] Z. Atcha *et al.*, "Cognitive enhancing effects of ghrelin receptor agonists.," *Psychopharmacology (Berl).*, vol. 206, no. 3,

pp. 415–27, Oct. 2009.

[132] S. P. Cahill, T. Hatchard, A. Abizaid, and M. R. Holahan, "An examination of early neural and cognitive alterations in hippocampal-spatial function of ghrelin receptor-deficient rats.," *Behav. Brain Res.*, vol. 264, pp. 105–15, May 2014.

[133] M. Kojima, H. Hosoda, Y. Date, M. Nakazato, H. Matsuo, and K. Kangawa, "Ghrelin is a growth-hormone-releasing acylated peptide from stomach.," *Nature*, vol. 402, no. 6762, pp. 656–60, Dec. 1999.

[134] M. A. Schalla and A. Stengel, "Molecular Sciences The Role of Ghrelin in Anorexia Nervosa," *Int. J. Mol. Sci.*, vol. 19, p. 2117, 2018.

[135] T. Reinehr, G. de Sousa, and C. L. Roth, "Obestatin and ghrelin levels in obese children and adolescents before and after reduction of overweight.," *Clin. Endocrinol. (Oxf).*, vol. 68, no. 2, pp. 304–10, Feb. 2008.

[136] P. Sumithran *et al.*, "Ketosis and appetite-mediating nutrients and hormones after weight loss," *Eur. J. Clin. Nutr.*, vol. 67, pp. 759–764, 2013.

[137] A. A. Gibson *et al.*, "Do ketogenic diets really suppress appetite? A systematic review and meta-analysis.," *Obes. Rev.*, vol. 16, no. 1, pp. 64–76, Jan. 2015.

[138] S. B. Sondike, N. Copperman, and M. S. Jacobson, "Effects of a low-carbohydrate diet on weight loss and cardiovascular risk factor in overweight adolescents.," *J. Pediatr.*, vol. 142, no. 3, pp. 253–8, Mar. 2003.

[139] G. D. Foster *et al.*, "A randomized trial of a low-carbohydrate diet for obesity.," *N. Engl. J. Med.*, vol. 348, no. 21, pp. 2082–90, May 2003.

[140] C. W. Shih, M. E. Hauser, L. Aronica, J. Rigdon, and C. D. Gardner, "Changes in blood lipid concentrations associated with changes in intake of dietary saturated fat in the context of a healthy low-carbohydrate weight-loss diet: a secondary analysis of the Diet Intervention Examining The Factors Interacting with Treatment," *Am. J. Clin. Nutr.*, vol. 109, no. 2, pp. 433–441, Feb. 2019.

[141] C. Kosinski and F. R. Jornayvaz, "Effects of Ketogenic Diets on Cardiovascular Risk Factors: Evidence from Animal and Human Studies.," *Nutrients*, vol. 9, no. 5, May 2017.

[142] P. J. Cox *et al.*, "Nutritional Ketosis Alters Fuel Preference and Thereby Endurance Performance in Athletes.," *Cell Metab.*, vol. 24, no. 2, pp. 256–68, 2016.

[143] A. C. Goldhamer *et al.*, "Medically Supervised Water-Only Fasting in the Treatment of Borderline Hypertension," 2002.

[144] E. S. Gordon, M. Goldberg, and G. J. Chosy, "A New Concept in the Treatment of Obesity: A 48-hour total fast followed by six meals a day and later by stepwise increases in food and calorie intake has permitted patients to lose weight that they show no tendency to regain for periods of up to 6 months. It also promoted spontaneous evolution of good dietary habits.," *JAMA*, vol. 186, no. 1, pp. 50–60, Oct. 1963.

[145] T. J. THOMSON, J. RUNCIE, and V. MILLER, "Treatment of obesity by total fasting for up to 249 days.," *Lancet*, vol. 2, pp. 992–996, 1966.

[146] D. A. Fraser *et al.*, "A Preliminary Study of Circadian Serum Cortisol Concentrations in Response to a 72-hour Fast in Rheumatoid Arthritis Patients not Previously Treated with Corticosteroids," *Clin. Rheumatol.*, vol. 20, no. 2, pp. 85–87, Mar. 2001.

[147] "Debinking Detox," 2009. [Online]. Available: https://web.archive.org/web/2014041809143 9/http://www.senseaboutscience.org/pages/de bunking-detox.html.

[148] A. Michalsen *et al.*, "Original Article · Originalarbeit Metabolic and Psychological Response to 7-Day Fasting in Obese Patients with and without Metabolic Syndrome," 2013.

[149] H. Lützner and F. W. de Toledo, "Fasten als Erlebnis, medizinische Prävention und Therapie," in *Ernährung und Fasten als Therapie*, Berlin, Heidelberg: Springer Berlin Heidelberg, 2010, pp. 167–198.

[150] J. F. Trepanowski, R. E. Canale, K. E. Marshall, M. M. Kabir, and R. J. Bloomer, "Impact of caloric and dietary restriction regimens on markers of health and longevity in humans and animals: a summary of available findings.," *Nutr. J.*, vol. 10, p. 107, Oct. 2011.

[151] K. A. Varady and M. K. Hellerstein, "Alternate-day fasting and chronic disease prevention: a review of human and animal trials.," *Am. J. Clin. Nutr.*, vol. 86, no. 1, pp. 7–13, Jul. 2007.

[152] C. Oleaga, C. J. Ciudad, V. Noé, and M. Izquierdo-Pulido, "Coffee polyphenols change the expression of STAT5B and ATF-2 modifying cyclin D1 levels in cancer cells," *Oxid. Med. Cell. Longev.*, vol. 2012, p. 390385, 2012.

[153] F. Pietrocola *et al.*, "Coffee induces autophagy in vivo," *Cell Cycle*, vol. 13, no. 12, pp. 1987–1994, Jun. 2014.

[154] N. Zhao, X. Zhang, C. Song, Y. Yang, B. He, and B. Xu, "The effects of treadmill exercise on autophagy in hippocampus of APP/PS1 transgenic mice," *Neuroreport*, vol. 29, no. 10, pp. 819–825, Jul. 2018.

[155] E. Ferraro, A. M. Giammarioli, S. Chiandotto, I. Spoletini, and G. Rosano, "Exercise-Induced Skeletal Muscle Remodeling and Metabolic Adaptation: Redox Signaling and Role of Autophagy," *Antioxid. Redox Signal.*, vol. 21, no. 1, pp. 154–176, Jul. 2014.

[156] P. F. Finn and J. F. Dice, "Ketone Bodies Stimulate Chaperone-mediated Autophagy," *J. Biol. Chem.*, vol. 280, no. 27, pp. 25864–25870, Jul. 2005.